The Mullet:

Hairstyle of the Gods

Larson / Hoskyns

The Mullet
Hairstyle of the Gods

Mark Larson / Barney Hoskyns

with illustrations by Maria Burgaleta Larson

BLOOMSBURY

First published in Great Britain 1999
by Bloomsbury Publishing Plc
38 Soho Square, London W1D 3HB

Text design and copyright © 1999 Mark Larson and Barney Hoskyns

The moral right of the authors has been asserted

A CIP catalogue record for this book
is available from the British Library

ISBN 0 7475 4424 7

10 9 8 7

Concept by Mark Larson and Barney Hoskyns
Design and art direction by Mark Larson

Text image generation by Mark Larson Design
Studio Photography by Jennifer Levy and Les Morsillo

Printed and bound in Hong Kong / China by South China Printing Co

Thank you...

Some gave all: Maria Burgaleta Larson and Victoria Sandler for innumerable contibutions to both text and artwork

Some gave a great deal: Jennifer Levy, Les Morsillo

Some gave really quite a lot: Jake and Fred Hoskyns, Iris and Emma Larson, Barry Price and April Traum, Liz Caprotti, Happy and Jane Traum, Dennis Collins, Andy Weitzer and Elysa London, Matt Caprotti, Chris Bailey, Kyle Bailey, Gene Burgaleta, Ian Worpole, Ursula and Emma Worpole, Ilana Weiss, Sean and Connor Ritchey, Matthew Hamilton and Mike Jones at Bloomsbury, Julian Alexander at LAW, Simon and Suzy Frith, Bruce Taylor, Jonathon Green, Daniel Gilson at Dan's Mullet Haven, Mark Maiocco and Mike Reinwald, J.R. Rost, Eddie Vedder, Colleen Combs, Mark Grunblatt, Jack Morelli, Michelle Butnick Press, Nancy Glowinski and Eric Smalkin at Gamma Liaison (New York), Mark Extance and Glen Marks at Rex Features (London), Peter Orlowsky at Allsport (New York)

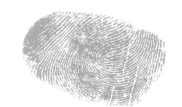

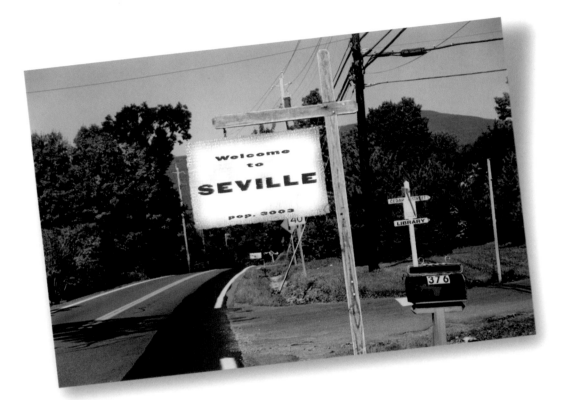

Welcome
to
SEVILLE
pop. 3003

376

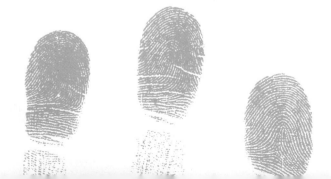

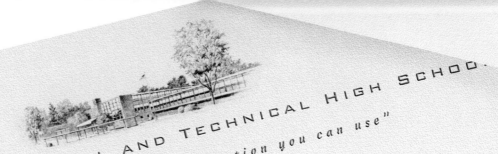

THE SEVILLE PRACTICAL AND TECHNICAL HIGH SCHOOL

"A practical education is an education you can use"

Dear Mrs. Dunkelschwester,

It falls, once again, to me as principal of The Seville Practical and Technical High School, a school, may I add, with a long tradition of providing a definitely "above average" education to the young people of the tri-town area, to address this, the latest affront to the moral standard and social moire of the community at large and to our student body and faculty specifically. As usual, this involves your son, Lincoln. While I have no desire to quash the "creative spirit," and far be it from me to "dictate" the "right" and "wrong" of something so personal, when it comes to matters of personal hygiene I expect that you will understand when I tell you that in a society the individuals must bend slightly to accommodate the good of the whole. A certain individual, and I think you know who I mean, has, quite a "stir." Freedom is fine but this hair thing has gotten out of hand and I simply must put my foot down. As a school official one tries to do the best one can but then one is simply not listened to and one's things are glued to one's desk and such...well you can see it would get to one can't you? I will expect you and your son in my office Monday at 9AM if you can find him and wake him at that hour. Please tell him that in school pants are not optional attire. Oh, and I'm serious. I want ALL of the hubcaps back.

Sincerely,

Dunton P. Peavey

Dunton P. Peavey, Principal

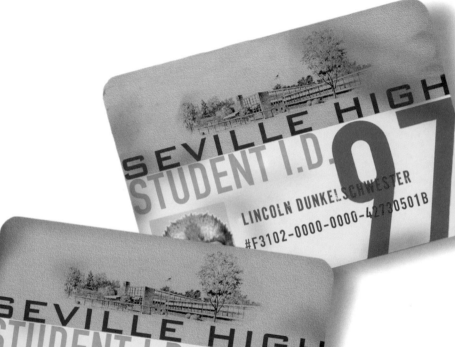

SEVILLE HIGH
STUDENT I.D. 07
LINCOLN DUNKELSCHWESTER
#F3102-0000-0000-42730501B

SEVILLE HIGH
STUDENT I.D. 07
THEODORE NUGENT FACHNAGEL
#F3102-0000-0000-42730500B

"The study of hair, I found out, does *not* take you to the superficial edge of our society, the place where everything silly and insubstantial must dwell. It takes you, instead, to the centre of things."

Grant McCracken,
Big Hair: A Journey into the Transformation of Self (1995)

＊

"Almost every male who paid the $3 cover charge wore his hair in that mysteriously durable style – still ubiquitous after years of hipster mockery – short in front, long in back, and known variously as a "Mullet", a "Trans Am", a "short-long", or a "neckwarmer". I had heard of only one ironic Mullet in my entire life, but the sight of so many of them in one place made me confront the possibility that the entire male population of Fort Wayne were born ironists and miles ahead of Yum-Yum in the commentary-on-the-tastes-of-middle-America competition."

Thomas Frank, "Pop Music in the Shadow of Irony",
Harper's, March 1998

MULLET MENU

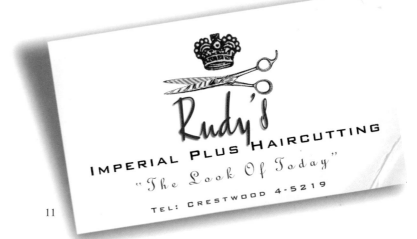

11

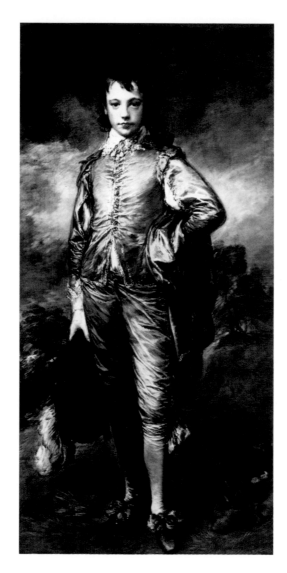

Gainsborough's Blue Mullet Boy

PROLOGUE

"One on the sides, don't touch the back,
Six on the top and don't cut it wack, Jack..."

The Beastie Boys, *"Mullet Head" (1994)*

They are everywhere you look. They are short at the front and long in the back. They are Mullets, and they rule.

Maybe you have a third cousin with a Mullet, or maybe it's just the skinny dude who fills up your car at the local gas station. Maybe it's the enormo-bottomed roadie you saw humping gear at that Garbage gig the other day.

You won't see many Mullets in London or Manhattan, or in a lot of other supposedly cool places. They don't often appear on MTV. But you'll see them in the suburbs, and in the heartlands. They're all over Latin America and eastern Europe.

No one seems entirely sure whence the term "Mullet" derives. Does Billy Ray Cyrus look like a fish? Not really. Yet you have to admit that the word sounds right. Perhaps it is connected to the old French word *mulet*, meaning "dim", or to the heraldic term "Mullets of the Field". "The best I can offer is the 19th century slang 'Mullethead', meaning a fool," says slang lexicographer Jonathon Green. "I can only assume that the hairstyle is some kind of anthropomorphic take on the fish." Note, however, that the second edition of *Webster's New International Dictionary* (1932) gives a definition of "mullet" as a verb meaning "to curl or dress the hair".

Membership of the unspoken brotherhood of Mullet-lovers includes such *cognoscenti* of outlandish tonsure as Evan Dando and Fountains of Wayne, although nobody has done more to champion the Mullet than the three amigos who comprise primo hip hop act the Beastie Boys. Not content with releasing the seminal "Mullet Head" on the B-side of their 1994 single "Sure Shot", Ad-Rock, MCA and Mike D dedicated several pages of their splendid magazine *Grand Royal* to what was until now the single most scholarly treatise on the Mullet ever published. For his pioneering field work amongst the aspiring guitar heroes of Hollywood, *Grand Royal* poobah Mike D surely merits inclusion in the future Mullet Hall of Fame. (Current favoured sites: Dusseldorf, Peoria, Hartlepool.)

Consider for a moment that the following have all sported Mullets of one description or another: David Bowie, Bono, Lou Reed, Link Ray, Paul McCartney, Roberto Baggio, Chris Waddle,

Andre Agassi, Mel Gibson, Barry White, Ice T, Eazy E, Eric Idle, Suzi Quatro, and Larry Fortensky. Gaze on that pantheon, ye mortals, and tremble.

"For some it's an endless debate, for others no question," writes Mimi Pond in her *Splitting Hairs: The Bald Truth About Bad Hair Days* (1998). "Should I wear it long or short? If it's long, it may just lay there like a Portuguese man-of-war on your head, limp and slack, [but] if it's short, is it just a copout?" With a few deft snips of the scissors, the Mullet solves Pond's problem in one, for its genius lies simply in the opportunity it affords one to become two people: someone who from the front looks like a regular person, but who from the back is an untamed party animal-cum-guitar hero-cum-Viking warrior. Party on!

From surfers to ski bums, stock-car racers to soap-opera stars, wrestlers to Roger Clinton, the Mullet has come to dominate the coiffure of America's soft white blue-collar underbelly. "To me," opines Beastie Boys acolyte The Captain, "the Mullet is as American as pick-ups with rifle racks, tractor pulls, Wal-Mart, wet T-shirt contests, slapping your girl upside the head with a frying pan and living in the woods."

The Captain is right, though he omits to mention the hairstyle's universality – the fact that its impact has been felt in every corner of our planet, among all God's peoples. If *Grand Royal* was correct in surmising that the Mullet had become "the ultimate Woodstock II 'do" – "New Wave on top, a bit b-boy on the sides, rock steady in back" – then we have to acknowledge that "Woodstock" (and yes, even "Woodstock II") has itself become a global mindset, as much a part of the lives of Australians, Filipinos, Swedes, Bolivians, Koreans, and Montenegrans as of hip young Americans. One world, one love, one hairstyle...

"I had a crew cut when I was really young, but it showed too much face," Mullethead Scotty Bugatti told *Grand Royal*. "I had long hair when I was in high school, but it got in my eyes." Now Scotty combines the best of both worlds, commanding his Queens barber to "spike the top but don't touch the back". The result is a glorious example of the outer-borough Italian-American Mullet known as the Guido. "The advantages are that it keeps my neck warm and impresses chicks with big hair. And with work, if my hair was long and all one length I wouldn't be taken as seriously."

Has anyone ever put the case for the Mullet so eloquently? Scotty, here's lookin' at you, kid.

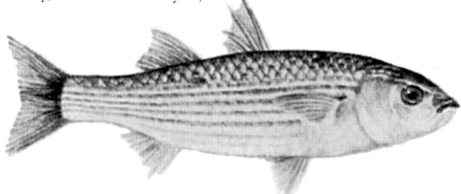

The
SPOON & BOWL
DINER
We may not be neat but we're fast!

TABLE	GUESTS	CHECK NO.	SERVER
		401155	

hamburger and fries $2.75

I CAN ONLY SAY THAT I WAS
VERY HUNGRY AN THAT IS
WHAT MADE ME DO IT.
P.S. YOUR FRIES R
THE BEST IN TOWN.
ALSO, YOU MAY WANT
TO CLOSE THE
BATHROOM WINDOW
OR EVERYBODY WILL
GO OUT THAT WAY.
LINK D.

4550

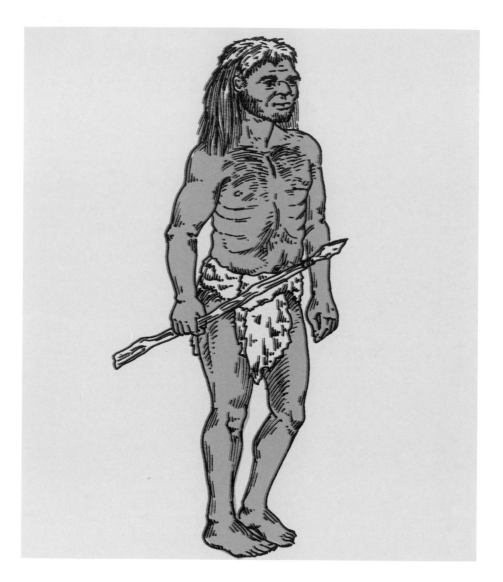

[Figure 1]

ROOTS

"Hair is just there as a product of our biological inheritance; but it cannot be just left there. Hair must be dealt with..."

Gananath Obeyesekere,
Hair: Its Power and Meaning in Asian Cultures

Let's face it, human civilization has spawned some amazing haircuts over the millenia. Since time immemorial, people have curled, permed, chopped, frizzed, streaked, and baked their hair into fabulous shapes. So it should come as no great surprise that the Mullet has appeared in prototype form in several cultures.

In fact, if artists' impressions are anything to go by, the original or *ur*-Mullet dates all the way back to the dawn of human civilisation. Depictions of Neanderthal Man as a scantily-clad savage with an unmistakably short-on-top-but-long-and-scraggly-at-the-back 'do [FIGURE 1] may explain the popularity of "Ape Drape" as one of the Mullet's many synonyms.

It seems likely that man's first tentative experiments in the field of depilation were prompted first and foremost by pragmatic

[FIGURE 2]

considerations: above all, the need to keep the hair out of the eyes while simultaneously allowing it to grow long at the back for the purposes of insulating the neck (hence another common synonym, "the Neck Blanket"). Thus do the Mullet's roots run deep through the collective unconscious of *homo sapiens*, explaining why the style has never gone completely out of so-called "fashion".

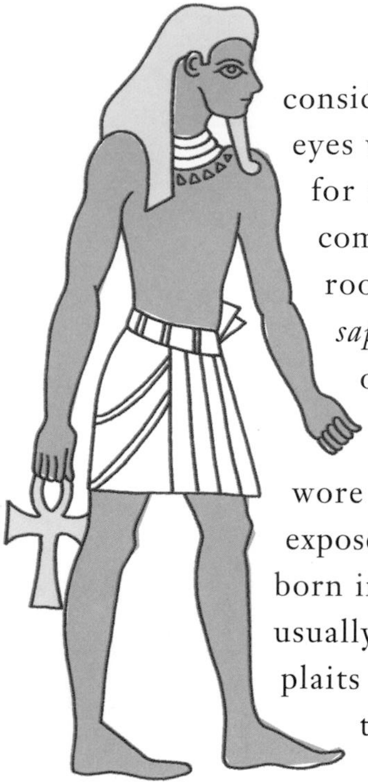

Although early tribes like the Hittites and Moabites wore their hair in elaborate styles that left the ears pointedly exposed, one would have to say that the first real Mullet was born in ancient Egypt [FIGURE 2]. True, the Egyptian Mullet was usually a wig made of black wool or flax, woven or braided into plaits (poor Egyptians had to make do with felt). Nonetheless the Mulletular design of these wigs leaves no doubt as to the aesthetic intentions of the people who wore them. Cut short over the scalp, where it precisely followed the contours of the wearer's head, the Egyptian Mullet dropped dramatically to the shoulders, where the flaxen strands parted, flowing simultaneously down the back and upper chest. Nor was it just Egyptian men who wore wigs: the Lady or "Fe-Mullet" almost certainly has its origins in this period [FIGURE 3], doubtless explaining why it is so often referred to as "the Sphinx".

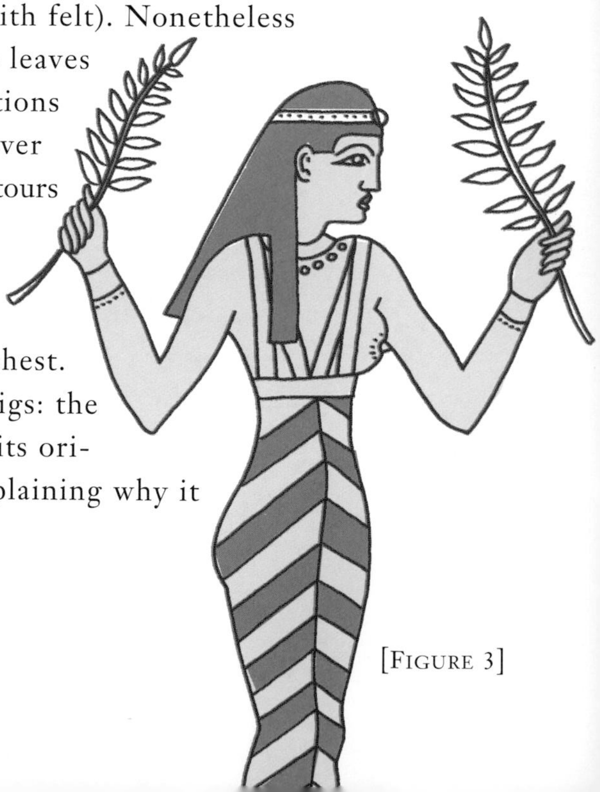

20

[FIGURE 3]

A little later, the Assyrians grew their thick, bristly hair long, although they too wore wigs. Coupled with their long, often artificial, beards, the Assyrian Mullet was highly ornamental – layered, with straight hair culminating in knots of curls [FIGURE 4]. The Persians wore their hair shorter than the Assyrians, although if anything the bi-level effect of the Persian Mullet was even more pronounced, with the top consisting of tousled curls and the bottom fanning out across the shoulders in long braided ringlets [FIGURE 5]. Talk about two-fer-the-price-of-one...

[FIGURE 4]

Rather less ornamental was the Celtic Mullet [FIGURE 6]. The Celts made little effort on the hairdressing front, but they did tend to thin out the sides of their shaggy mops while letting them droop down to the nape. Ancestor of legions of modern-day bikers, wrestlers, and heavy metal drummers, the Celtic Mullethead famously dyed his hair with green and blue woad. Nice one, McFergus!

[FIGURE 5]

The ancient Greeks flirted with the Mullet, braiding their locks into long ringlets that they tucked behind their ears, but after the Persian Wars of the early 5th century B.C., young Athenian males lopped off their Mullets and consecrated them to the gods.

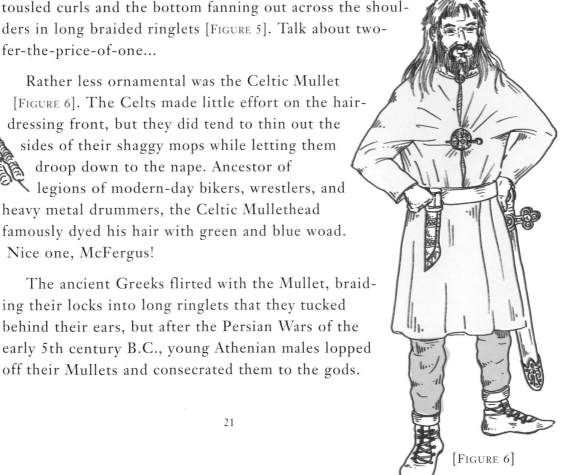

[FIGURE 6]

21

Thus was born the short classical hairstyle we know from the famous statues of the period, a style which spoke volumes about the Greek equation of long hair with disordered emotions. It was left to Greek women to keep the Mullet alive, in the form of artificial curls on top and long braided hair drawn into a knot at the back (often dyed blonde).

Like the Greeks, the Romans were hostile to the Mullet, even going so far as to snip the tresses of the male barbarians they conquered. For the most part, Roman men brushed their hair forward from the crown and left it severe at the back, with optional laurel leaves worn to conceal baldness. (It is hard, it must be said, to imagine Julius Caesar with a Mullet.) After the fall of the Roman Empire, however, the cut made a comeback: both the Visigoths and the Vikings anticipated the thuglike demeanour and follicular deportment of the average American football player by well over a thousand years.

The Merovingian period in France (481-752) was no friendlier to the Mullet than the Greek or Roman eras had been. Men wore plaited hair atop their scalps but cut the back of their hair. (Check out Charlemagne, for example.) The Saxons of the 9th and 10th centuries also wore their locks on the short side, combed forward from the crown and brushed back from the forehead. The Normans were more extreme still, fashioning the first genuine Anti-Mullet by shaving the backs of their heads in a primitive kind of pudding-bowl [FIGURE 7].

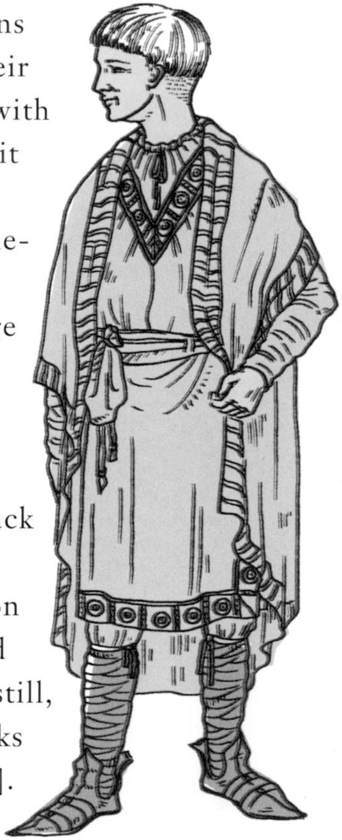

22

[FIGURE 7]

Shoulder-length hair parted on either side with the front in a fringe became popular in the 12th century, though the ears tended to be covered. Short hair was back in by the 14th century, brushed forward at the sides and rolled under. Bowl-shaped cuts remained fashionable till about 1460, largely owing to high *carcaille* collars that fitted all the way up the neck. In medieval France, Joan of Arc had a pudding bowl, and the fact was rightly held against her: a Mullet might have saved her life. (Significantly, the pudding bowl never took root in Germany, where the modern Mullet has flourished.) Around 1465, collars became shorter and a long, Mullet-style pageboy cut became all the rage, its curled shape kept in place with resins and egg white [FIGURE 8]. Yummy!

In the early 16th century, hair was generally worn shoulder-length, often with a fringe, but in the 1560s it became fashionable for men to cut it close to the scalp, brushing it up into bristles that were held in place with gum. Then, once again, length and elaborateness were the order of the day, with lovelocks falling poetically to the shoulders. The English Civil War of the following century would be remembered as much for hairstyles as for issues of monarchy and republicanism: the Royalists wore long curly hair while the "roundheads" favoured austere, puritanical crops. Sadly, no one thought to revive the Mullet as an aesthetic/political compromise.

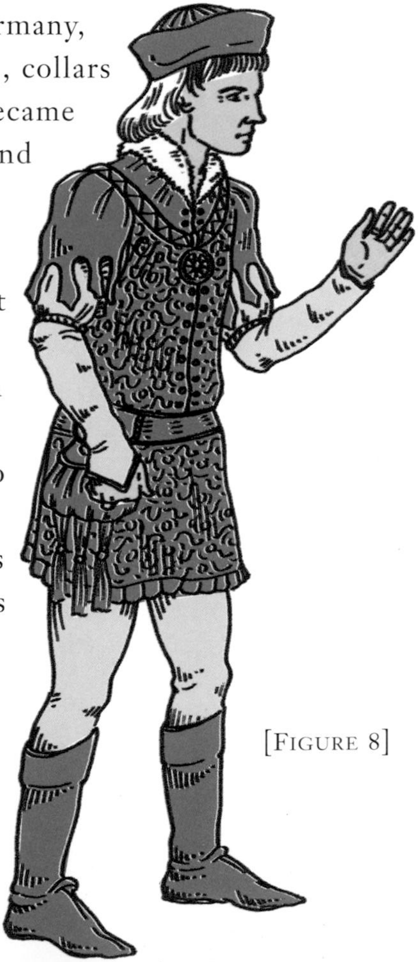

[FIGURE 8]

23

Far from England, meanwhile, the Manchu conquest of China had profound and long-lasting consequences for hair. Traditionally, Chinese men had worn their hair long and bound-up, but from 1644 onwards they were required to shave their foreheads and plait their hair in elongated braids that dangled to neck level – a style known as the *queue*. "Keep your head, lose your hair; keep your hair, lose your head" was the rather sinister advice of the Qing Dynasty, which persecuted hair-growers mercilessly. (Centuries later, with the 1911 uprising against the Manchus, *queue* cutting became a major political issue.) It should be pointed out that while the *queue* was a Mullet of sorts, it was in reality an abuse of the Mullet – a travesty rooted in the obsessive need to control.

Back in Blighty, the reign of Charles II saw the birth of the periwig, usually made of goat or horse hair, though sometimes fashioned from human tresses. In France, too, the wig came to dominate the coiffure of the *beau monde*. When Louis XIII lost his hair around 1633, wigs replaced the flowing locks of the early 17th century. By the 18th century, wigs grew to fantastical proportions, and came in myriad bizarre shapes. Not until the era of heavy metal "poodle" cuts would humanity again witness the rococo excesses of periwigged Europe. Inevitably, perhaps, a reaction against all things powdered and perfumed set in: by the century's end the wigs had become notably shorter, tied back with ribbons and leaving most of the ear exposed.

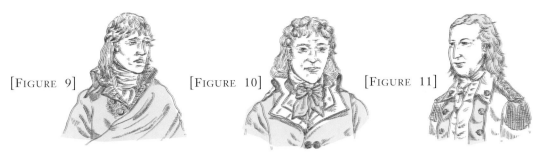

[FIGURE 9]   [FIGURE 10]   [FIGURE 11]

Only when wigs were finally abandoned in the late 18th century did the Mullet make a proper comeback. But what a comeback it was! Surely no hairstyle could have been better suited to the romantic, radical spirit of the times. Starting with Napoleon Bonaparte [FIGURE 9] and the revolutionaries of Paris (Camille Desmoulins, [FIGURE 10]), the "Romantic" Mullet was as likely to be seen on the head of an American general like Horatio Gates [FIGURE 11] as cascading down the neck of a poet like Samuel Taylor Coleridge. After the excessive formality and pompous opulence of wigs, here at last were real men, their unkempt hair cut with a deliberate disregard for neatness and all of a piece with their dishevelled clothing. Even young Parisian blades who had opposed the French revolution were now seen with bi- (or even multi-) level hair hanging lankly about their heads, while paintings such as Gainsborough's *Blue Boy* suggest that the Mullet was the preferred hairstyle among privileged English youth.

"Loose hair for mature men was usually a public virile ornament," writes Anne Hollander in *Sex and Suits*; "[it was] akin to the display of muscle and stature, a sign of sexual force in action." The robust sexuality of young revolutionaries and Romantic poets has never

25

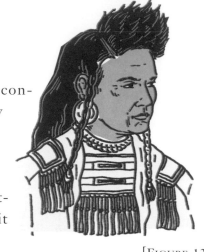

[FIGURE 12]

been in question, but only now can we make the connection between their political and literary potency and the sheer virility of the Mullet. It may also be worth noting here that the Mullet has always been in vogue among Native Americans [FIGURE 12], and that the likes of Buffalo Bill Cody liked nothing better than to keep things tidy out front while letting it all hang out behind him [FIGURE 13].

It should come as no great surprise that, with the onset of the repressive Victorian era, the Mullet began once again to fade from view. By the mid-19th century, curls and waves were in vogue, but thanks to a new taste for high collars men began to wear their hair shorter at the back than in front. With the focus now on outsize moustaches and side whiskers – "Mutton Chops", "Dundrearys", and "Piccadilly Weepers" – this was not a propitious time for the Mullet.

Little was to change over the next hundred years. By the early 20th century, male hair was shorter than it had ever been: the "short back and sides" so beloved of military disciplinarians was now ubiquitous in civilian life. Between the two World Wars, there was a brief vogue for the Pompadour, with the hair slightly raised in front, but that was about it.

Not until the rock era did the Mullet reclaim its rightful place on the world's stage. It took an androgynous, carrot-haired starman to usher it into the bosom of popular culture.

26

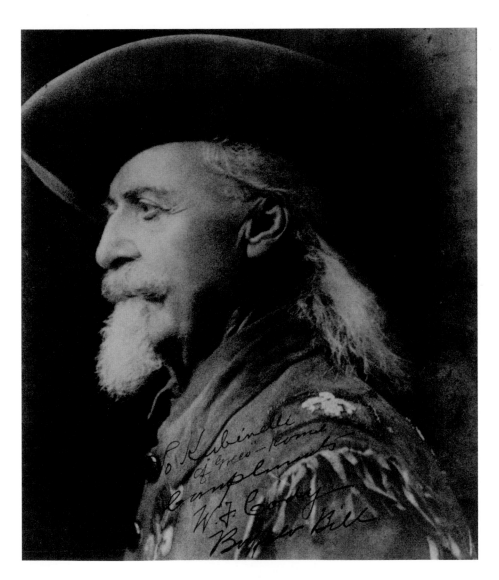

[FIGURE 13]

THIS DUDE RULES!

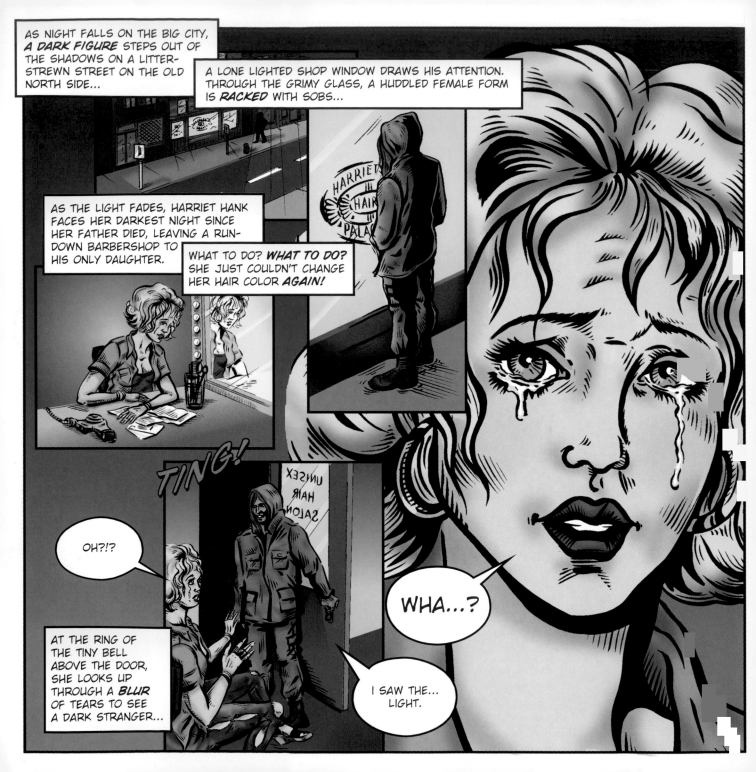

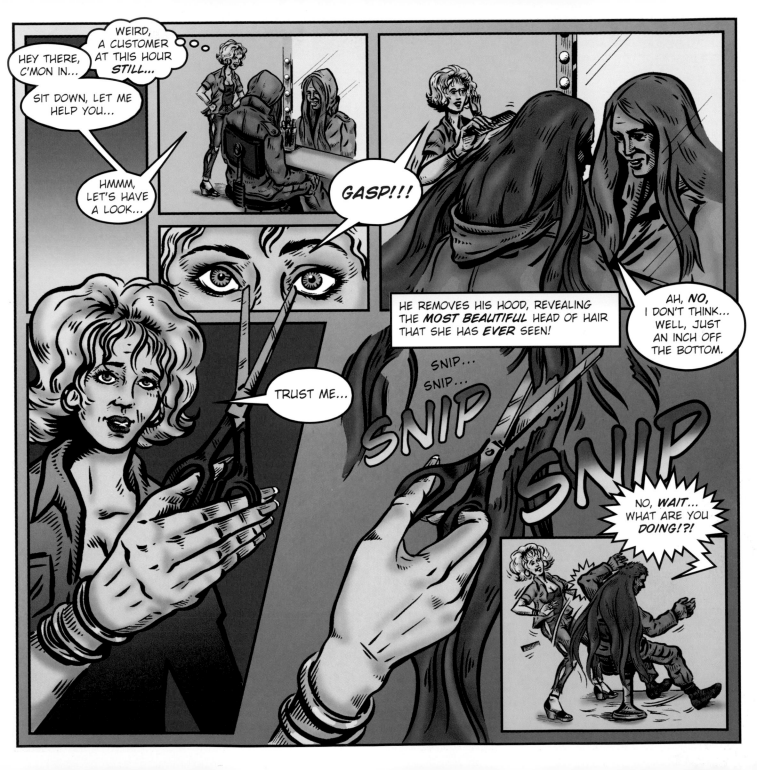

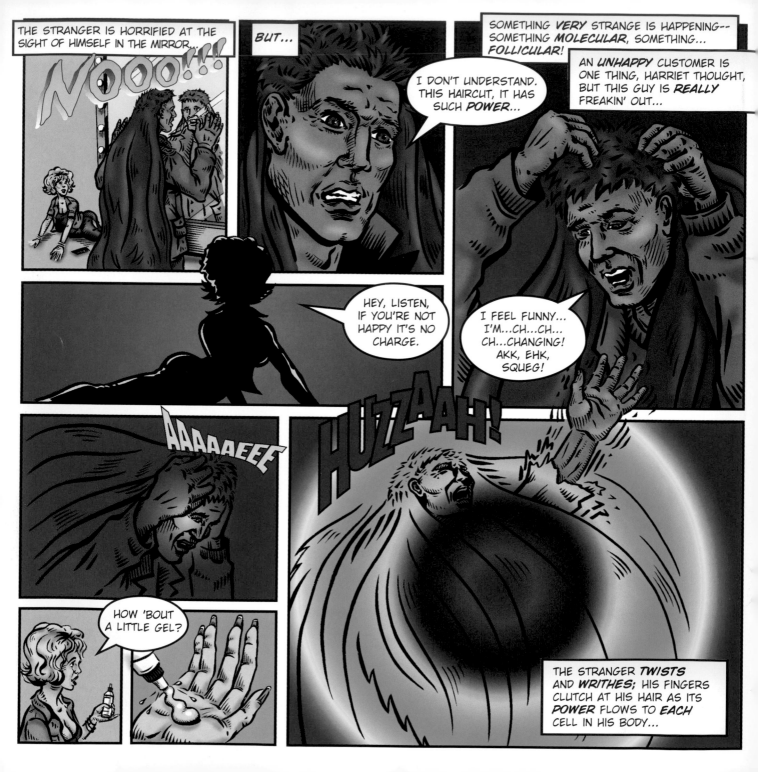

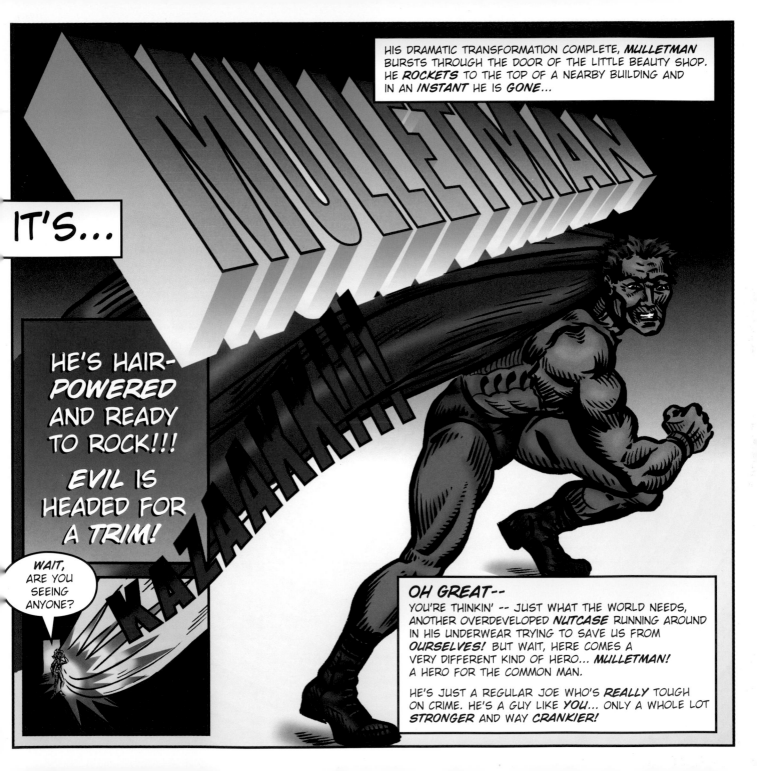

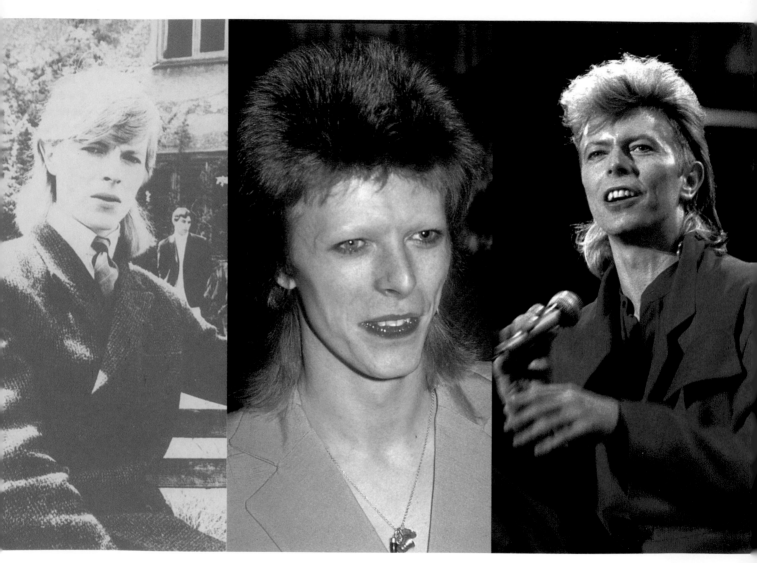

Three ages of a bi-level superstar: David Bowie in '65, '73 & '87

GROWTH

"Hair are your aerials."

Danny, *Withnail and I*

Significantly, David Bowie had already experimented with a proto-Mullet back in his mod days as the lead singer of R&B combo the King Bees. A remarkable portrait of the then David Jones in 1965 shows a fey-looking youth with beautifully conditioned locks combed across his scalp, curling their way round his ears, and then re-emerging in radical collar-tickling tufts at least five inches long. Turns out the Thin White Duke was even more ahead of his time than we thought.

Several years later – early in 1972, to be precise – David Bowie was checking his long blond Veronica Lake tresses in the bedroom mirror one morning and decided he had to make more of a tonsorial statement to go with the birth of his new 'Ziggy Stardust' alter ego. His wife Angie had recently visited the Evelyn Paget salon on south London's Beckenham High Street, and had asked stylist Suzy Fossey to put stripes – red, white, and blue – in her hair. Satisfied that Fossey was on their fashion wavelength, Angie asked her to come to the Bowies' flat.

33

"D'you like the way my hair's been cut?" Bowie inquired of Fossey when the stylist came by.

"Not really," she replied. "It's boring. Everyone's got a long shag these days."

"What would *you* do, then?" Bowie asked.

"I'd have short hair, because no one's got short hair at the moment," said Suzy.

"I don't want any *ordinary* short cut," pouted Bowie reasonably.

Thus it was that Angie Bowie began leafing through some old copies of *Vogue* in search of inspiration. Half an hour later, with a small stroke of genius, this trio of trailblazers hit on a combination of two haircuts: a pointy front suggested by a picture in French *Vogue*, with the sides and back taken from two separate issues of German *Vogue*. It was a style that flew radically in the face of hippie modes: short and spiky on top, severe at the sides, but with long wisps trailing down the neck. It was the birth of the Rock Mullet as we know it, with the whole thing topped off by a shocking German dye called Red Hot Red.

In her autobiography *Backstage Passes*, Angie Bowie wrote that history was made that day – that the Ziggy Mullet was "the single most reverberant fashion statement of the '70s" – and she wasn't wrong. When the Bowies sashayed into their favourite gay club

LIKE, YOUR HAIR IS YOUR STATEMENT— IT SAYS WHAT YOU CAN'T THINK OF SAYING!
— LINK DUNKELSCHWESTER

34

that night, it wasn't just the queens who drooled. "I don't think I'm outrageous," Bowie told the *Daily Express* the following week. "It's just a more exciting way of looking."

The influence of the Ziggy Mullet may not have been immediate, but thousands of Bowie boys and girls were soon following suit. As with all avant-garde phenomena, it took a while for the style to percolate through to the mainstream, and most male rockers still wore their hair in the basic androgynous, hair-over-the-ears shag style. Notwithstanding variants on the classic hippie-rock hairstyle like the Rod Stewart "rooster" cut, it was only when glam rock hit its stride that the Rock Mullet began to flourish properly. Some of the more splendid specimens of the time were those worn by Slade's goofy guitarist Dave Hill and Roxy Music's retro-Teddy Boy saxophonist Andy Mackay, the latter single-handedly defining the category of "Quiffed Mullet".

But it wasn't just glam rockers who seized upon the Mullet. Post-Beatles, Paul McCartney was quick to adopt the cut as the true style of rock'n'roll convenience. Meanwhile Linda, his wife and Wings bandmate, pioneered the "Fe-Mullet", a style seen before in somewhat muted form on the heads of the sitcom stars Florence Henderson of *The Brady Bunch* and Suzanne Pleshette of *The Bob Newhart Show*.

Nobody, however, could have foreseen the Mullet explosion of the 1980s, a decade in which the short-long compromise cut infiltrated and took over the worlds of rock music, sport, fashion, and pornography. Some would say that a watershed moment was Rush's Geddy Lee unveiling his Canadian Prog-Rock Mullet during a five-night stand at New York's Radio City Music Hall in September 1983. In fact, the Mullet would become popular amongst a wide variety of American rock bands, from proggers to hard rockers to AOR noodlers: Journey's Steve Perry, REO Speedwagon's Kevin Cronin, Styx's Tommy Shaw, Loverboy's Mike Reno, and GTR's Max Bacon all sported Mullets at various points in the '80s. None of those dudes, though, could have held a candle to Klaus Meine of German metal monsters the Scorpions. (How about those krauts!)

Mullets also began to blossom in the British "New Romantic" community, most spectacularly on the heads of pin-up idols like Nik Kershaw, Duran Duran's John Taylor, and Kajagoogoo's Limahl. (Note that the 'goos' Nick Beggs single-headedly birthed the very fetching Braided Mullet.) Regrettably, contemporaries Haircut 100 failed to include a single Mullet in their lineup, but most great '80s bands – from Talk Talk to Tears For Fears – boasted at least one bi-leveller in their ranks.

In the Big Hair '80s, when it was difficult to move for teased tresses and peroxide-blonde manes, the Modern Rock Mullet was an essential video-pop cut, ubiquitous on MTV. Daryl Hall and John Oates had Mullets. The Cars had Mullets. Richard Marx and Michael Bolton had Mullets. Bono, in his Red Rocks/*Under a Blood Red Sky* phase, sported the haircut that had not yet dared to speak its name. By the end of the decade, even Lou Reed was wearing one – perhaps the most magnificent Rock Mullet ever worn by a punk godfather.

Let us not forget the giant contribution made to the Rock Mullet's growth by the Session Bassist. In the past, bass players had tended to be either excessively hirsute (Leland Sklar) or completely hairless (Tony Levin). With the elevation of the "picker" to superstar status in the '80s, however, the Mullet came to the rescue, transforming countless unsung worker bees in Nashville and LA into bi-level heroes of The Axe That Hath But Four Strings. (Raise your glasses to Mike Chapman, Hutch Hutchinson, Dave Pomeroy, Neil Stubenhaus, and so many, many more...)

And that's far from all, folks. In the '80s, tennis players wore Mullets: Pat Cash, Andre Agassi, Martina Navratilova. Movie stars wore Mullets: Mel Gibson, Kurt Russell, Patrick Swayze. Soccer players wore Mullets: Roberto Baggio, Glenn Hoddle, Chris Waddle. Cricketers wore Mullets: Ian Botham, Alan Lamb, Geoff Thompson. American football players wore Mullets: Doug Flutie, Brian Bosworth, Golden Richards. Australian soap heart-throbs wore Mullets: Jason Donovan, Craig McLachlan. Hell, even *black* people wore Mullets: Barry White, Nicholas Ashford, the Rev. Al Sharpton.

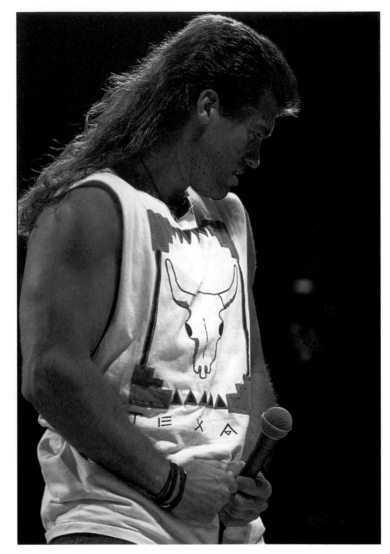

A Mullethead holds his own: Billy Ray Cyrus

Sports such as hockey, wrestling, and stock-car racing became especially fertile breeding grounds for the Mullet. Hockey players – particularly those with names ending in the letters "ic" – appeared to have been born with Mullets. By the end of the '80s, the cut was running riot through every mall, sports stadium and speedway in America. Worn with tight stonewashed jeans, sleeveless muscle T-shirts and mirrored sunglasses, the Mullet became a badge of pride, the hallmark of the rock'n'roll beer dude in his Camaro or Trans Am. Yet if you'd told the average Mullethead that he owed everything to a flame-haired rock'n'roll bisexual called Ziggy Stardust, he'd have smashed you over the head with a six-pack.

Only in the early '90s, after a soccer World Cup that treated the world to a feast of outlandish hairstyles from Eastern Europe and Latin A_____ ___ __ he term "Mullet" come into being. _____s are still scratching their heads as to _____ term, but etymology becomes irrelevant ___ el Bolton and Billy Ray Cyrus heave ____tive 1995 tract on *Homo Mulleticus* in ____ Mullet-spotting quickly became a ____ ockers. Motoring through Ohio and ___ our bus suddenly became an adventure

Dear Link,
your father and I
wish you would
reconsider this haircut
o_____
love,
Mom

39

The late '90s find the Mullet thriving in the domain of country music, with stars like Travis Tritt and Tracy Lawrence ill-concealing their manes beneath their Stetson hats. Rockers like Lou Reed and James Hetfield may have copped out and lopped off their locks, but celebs like Larry Fortensky are as committed to the cut as they ever were. There's a priceless Kid Mullet on *Home Improvement* (Zachary Ty Bryan), there's a Fe-Mulleted Lady Boxer (Christy Martin) and a MetroStars Latin Soccer Mullet (Marco Etcheverry). The Pittsburgh Penguins' Czech superstar Jaromir Jagr is keeping the Hockey Mullet alive and well into the new millenium. Every other baseball player in America seems to have what Joe Queenan quaintly refers to as "relief pitcher hair". Even *lesbians* like the Mullet.

The Mullet is the perfect 'do for the new millenium, a time when all the rules of personal appearance have been broken. "Once it was easy to tell a music act by its hair," writes Mimi Pond in *Splitting Hairs*. "Long hair – rock. Short hair meant something square, something Lawrence Welk-like. The Man. To youth, short hair was the problem, long hair the solution. These days, with the music industry exploding with all kinds of sounds, it's hard to tell who's on whose side." The Mullethead knows there are no "sides" anymore – that the Mullet is both *for* and *against*, *inside* and *outside*, *part of* and *apart from*. Indeed, one might almost argue that, from a psychoanalytical viewpoint, the Mullet is both

Ego (the short, neat top) and Id (the long, flowing back) – an analogy which extends into the realms of sex and sociology.

In his 1958 essay "Magical Hair", the anthropologist Edmund Leach suggested that in most cultures, long hair = unrestrained sexuality; short or partially shaved hair = restricted sexuality; and close-cropped hair = celibacy. Eleven years later, C.D. Hallpike countered with an essay entitled "Social Hair", which argued instead that long hair = being outside society, while short hair = re-entering society. In both cases, the has it both ways: his "short" hair withholds and c his "long hair" promises carnal joy and social r Gananath Obeyesekere is right that there seem oppositional dialectic" between loose hair and ha groomed or bound," then the Mullet has brough together. It's Apollo and Dionysus, Capitalism a Order and Disorder, Self and Other in one ma ambiguous crop.

Over a quarter-century since David Bowie Mullet continues to dazzle and delight – an e tamed fertility and regulated regeneration. For those about to "sho-lo", we salute you.

PRIVY PRANK

Speculation was widespread when it was discovered this morning that Omar Wiley's outhouse was sitting on top of the Fisherman's Bank & Trust Co. at 1445 North Main. When reached at the Dunk 'n' Roll, local police had no official comment other than to characterize the incident as a "prank." "You never know what will happen next," said Elizah Ball, waitress at The Spoon And Bowl Diner Fine Dining For All Occasions, "I'm thinking of locking my door." Eyewitness accounts were contradictory. Local businessman, Everette Clow of Clow Lumber, a fine place for all your wood and building needs, told this reporter, "He was running right at me so I got a good look, he was a big fella with a short haircut." But, Lyle Spingler of Spingler's Bait and Tackle said, "It was kinda dark but I saw him run down the side street and I can say for sure he had long hair." Once again, the peace of this quiet little upstate town has been shattered by what has become a pattern of mischief maisidnk.

Although the Mullet comes in a thousand and one shapes and forms – variations on a central sho-lo theme – there are a number of Mullet archetypes from which almost all other Mullets derive. It is true that some of these archetypes are ethnically determined, while others stem from specific activities or job descriptions. However, we offer them not as stereotypes or cartoons but as Platonic ideals, and as all the proof anyone could need of the Mullet's heartening universality. Far from being tied to certain demographics and socio-economic "groups", the Mullet's appeal has always transcended the barriers of race and class, uniting its wearers in a tacit, unspoken brotherhood. One might almost say that the Mullet is a kind of *fan hair for the common man* – a style that connects Michael Bolton not only to Martina Navratilova but to the Mullethead in the street. It is, quite simply, the great bi-leveller of our times.

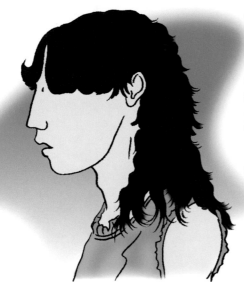

The Midwest Metal

A.K.A. *the Scorpion, the Bitchin' Vixen, the Hello Cleveland!*

The Free Bird of Planet Coiffure. From the rock halls to the mega-malls, this 'do is *de rigeur*. Best breeding grounds: truck stops, pool halls, rock clubs, body shops.

Vital accessories: Mirror shades, Muscle T-shirt, Gatorade, Velcro hi-tops, Satanic tats, pink guitar.

We're not worthy: Joe Elliott (Def Leppard), Dave Mustaine (Megadeth), Frank Beard (ZZ Top).

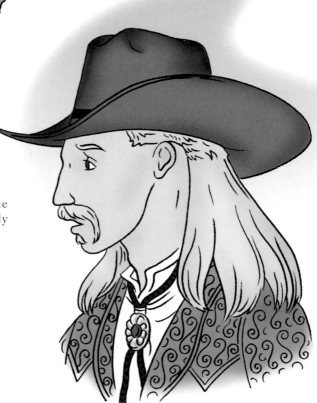

The Nashville

A.K.A. *the Twang'n'Go, the Achy Breaky, the Kentucky Waterfall*

Downhome and down your red neck, this is the essential cut for the cats in the hats. Fits neatly 'neath the Stetson and won't get in your eyes when you're downshiftin' the 18-wheeler.

Country Mullet Classic: Curly Pate & the Shag Band, "You Done Me Wrong (But I Won't Be Short For Long)" (1975).

Yee haw! Billy Ray Cyrus, Travis Tritt, Tracy Lawrence, Marty Stuart.

The Modern Rock

A.K.A. *the Pay to Play, the Backstage Pass, the Blade Runner*

Bike messenger by day, rock god by night, the Modern Rock Mullethead leaves a trail of mangled plectrums and bruised groupies in his dust. His band plays cyber-gothic techno-punk at the Coconut Teaszer. About to ink deal with Chernobyl Blowjob Records.

In Excess: John Taylor, the Psychedelic Furs, Ric Ocasek.

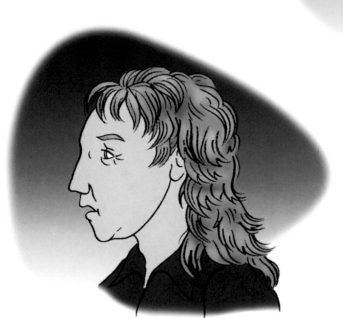

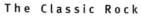

The Classic Rock

A.K.A. *the Drum Clinic, the Old Waver, the "Silver" Mullet*

Still bi-level after all these years, the Classic Rock Mullethead is found in every club, radio station, and record company on the planet. Still wears: Cure tour jacket. Still suffers from: "A&R man's cold". Still knows: he looks good.

Awright Mate! Paul McCartney, Geddy Lee, Jim Steinman.

The Relief Pitcher

A.K.A. *the Change-Up, the Benchwarmer, the Great White Hope*

Lean'n'mean, the relief pitcher's talent takes him from the trailer park to the major-league bull pen. As he strides to the mound in the bottom of the ninth, his flaxen mane flows from the back of his cap, every strand of hair gleaming with hope.

Strikeout! Randy Johnson, Mark Wohlers.

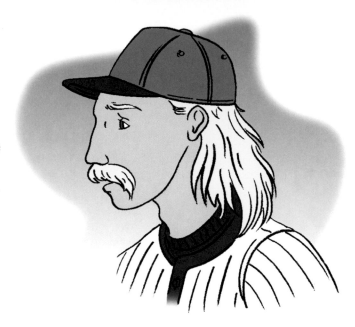

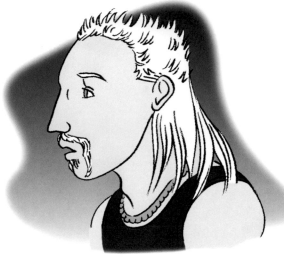

The Visigoth

A.K.A. *the Body Check, the Mauler, the Credible Hulk*

Sitting atop 300 lb of brawn and brew, the Visigoth is the Thor of the Mullet Universe. Where there is battle to be done – on canvas, gridiron, or ice – our boy is there, locks flying behind his helmet. (Remove teeth for full Hockey Mullet.)

Favourite haunts: Duluth, Toledo, Valhalla.

Crrrrunch! Brian Bosworth, Golden Richards.

The Latin Soccer Mullet

A.K.A. *the Libero, the "Diving Header", the Sudden Death*

There is no more fearsome sight than a tonsured Latin centre-forward rising to meet a pinpoint cross, his Mulleted tresses blinding the defenders around him. Essential *muleto* accessories: Gucci purse, lime-green Maserati, bottle-blonde spouse.

Golaaaazo!
Roberto Baggio,
Marco Etcheverry.

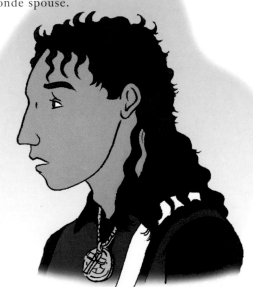

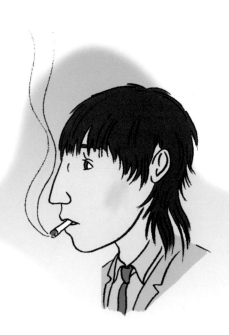

The Eastern Bloc

A.K.A. *"The Curtain"*,
the Prague Spring

The Mullet has long been
popular in Eastern Europe,
where its untrammelled
expressiveness and sheer flouting
of convention played a major role
in the fall of Soviet communism.
Surviving the collapse of the Berlin
wall, the Eastern Bloc *mulletkopf* remains
an eternal symbol of the struggle for freedom.

All the comrades sing: "Sweet Home Bratislava",
Heffy Spektrum (1987).

The English Mullet

A.K.A. *the Runt, the Castle
Donington, the Smokey Bacon*

Considering how vital the Mullet
has been to British culture –
from Samuel Taylor Coleridge
to Kajagoogoo – it's little wonder
that the cut lives on in the
heartland of Albion. Fertilised
by curry, Jagermeister lager, and
Embassy cigs, the English
Mullet stands tall in an uncertain
world, eschewing the ever-
changing fads of cool Brittania.

Best sightings: Northern discos,
fish'n'chip shops.

Eyup! Paul Calf, Tiger, Wicksy
on *EastEnders*.

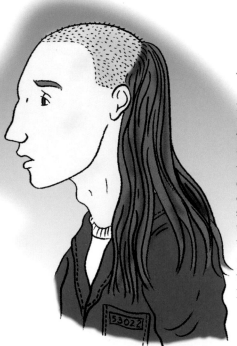

The Offender

A.K.A. *the Fringe Element*,
L'Etranger, *the Cape Fear*

The Offender is streetwear for
the street-aware. This Mullet
won't be "in your face" but lets
everybody know you won't back
down. Urban guerilla or big sky
survivalist, on the front line or
the chow line, you're ready to go
the distance.

You ain't seen me... right?
Wayne Lefaque, Billy Bob Wayne,
DeWayne X.

The Movie Star

A.K.A. *the Convertible, the Spago, the Lethal Weapon*

Always ready for the close-up, the "Holly-Mullet" trumpets buddy-buddy hijinks, transforming the everyday matinee idol into a death-defying *homme sauvage*. Ideal for car chases, love scenes, and any cinematic moment that requires a little extra in the back.

Lights, camera, action: Mel Gibson, Jean-Claude Van Damme, Kurt Russell, Patrick Swayze.

The Inspirational

A.K.A. *the Holy Roller, the True Believer, the Crown o'Thorns* [archaic]

Can we get a hallelujah for this beauty, and for every sanctified Mullethead sending out God's word to the people on America's cable stations? As it glistens in the kluge lights, the "Inspirational" reminds us of our trials on earth while reaching upwards to the heavens. Closer our scalps to thee...

The Power and the Glory: Brothers and sisters, get out your checkbooks – we don't get these hair products for free!

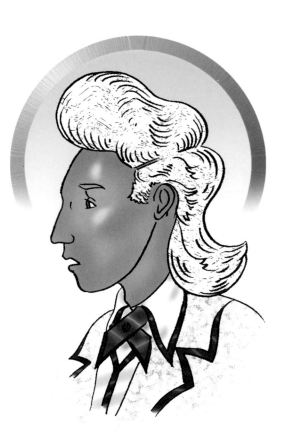

The African-American

A.K.A. *the Afro-Deeeeziak, the Black to the Phuture, the South Central Iced T*

The Mullet recognises no racial boundaries. From Jheri-curls to real fly girls, Lionel Richie to the Reverend Al Sharpton, the African-American screams soul, sex and sophistication from the heart of the black experience.

Shouts to the homies: Barry White, Buddy Guy, Nick Ashford, Steve Arrington.

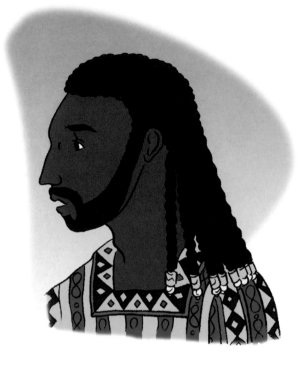

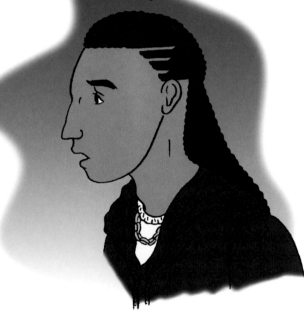

The Pan-Ethnic

A.K.A. *the Loverboy, the Hi-Lo Rider*

From Bay Ridge to El Segundo, the Hudson Bay to Tierra del Fuego, the Mullet is the "United Nations" of hairstyles – a multi-cultural 'do for every smooth-talking, cool-walking Casanova on the block. (Moustache advisable, gold chain mandatory.)

Yo! Guido, Chico, Rico, Nico, Paco, Dino, Singho...

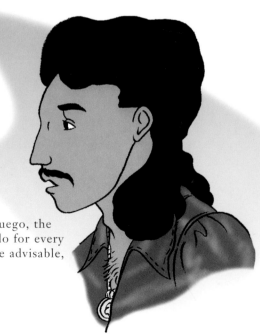

The Lady Mullet

A.K.A. *the Fe-Mullet, the Pleshette, the "Duck and Cover"*

The Mullet isn't just a guy thing, it's today's hairstyle for the woman on the go. From beach bunnies to biker chicks, jet-set superwomen to stressed-out soccer moms, ladies everywhere are enjoying the fruits of bi-level living. You've come a long way, baby!

Queen bees: Florence Henderson (*The Brady Bunch)*, Suzanne Pleshette (*The Bob Newhart Show*), Linda McCartney, Suzi Quatro, Sheena Easton.

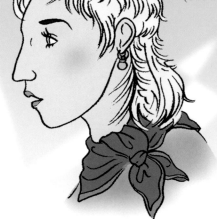

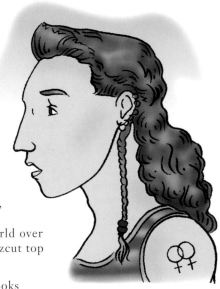

The Lesbian

A.K.A. *the Ripley, the Pallas Athene, the "WhaddaYOUlookinat?!"*

It's *really* not just a guy thing, as legions of butch gals the world over will attest. No style better suits the modern Amazon: the buzzcut top talks ♂, the flowing tail says ♀.

Lesbian Mullet Classic: Hairysmith Big Mambazos, "Lady Looks Like A Dude" (1994).

Taking back the highlights: Martina Navratilova, Indigo Girls.

The Executive

A.K.A. *the Weekend Warrior, the Gabardine Mangler, "Tha Playa"*

For the rebel with the washroom key, here is the ultimate dual-purpose, have-your-cake-and-eat-it hairstyle: short for when you face the boss, long for when you turn your back on society.

Essential accoutrement: motorcycle helmet in desk drawer.

Essential quote: "This is just my day gig."

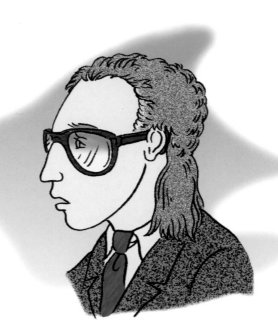

The Fading Glory

A.K.A. *the Bald Eagle, the* A La Recherche, *the Remains of the Day*

Why bid the Mullet *adieu* just because time has taken its toll on your scalp? Diehard dudes say No! What we lack on top we'll more than make up for in back. Let 'em know you'll still be standing when the party shuts down.

Key phrase: "I saw them live."

For old times' sake: Steve Stills, Michael Bolton, Hulk Hogan

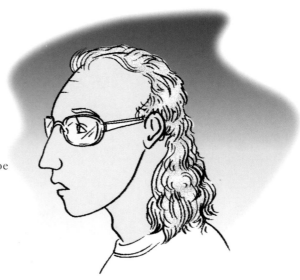

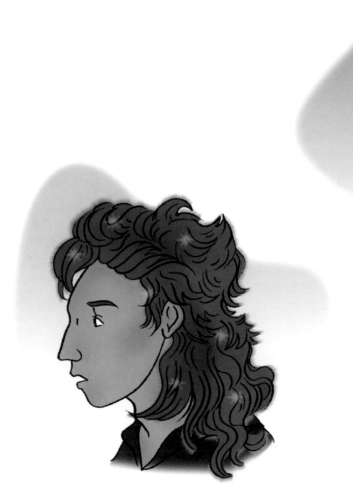

The Almost-Mullet

A.K.A. *the Quasi, the* Faux, *the Equivocal*

It's a pitiful sight: men and women who lack the courage of their convictions, curbing the natural impulse to let their hair down. Who do these folks think they're kidding? As Eric Clapton said , "In the sun, rain, and snow/let it flow, let it flow..."

For shame! Jerry Seinfeld, Penn Jillette, Latrell Sprewell.

The Mullet Deluxe

A.K.A. *the Fountainhead, the* Pelo Grande, le bouffant extraordinaire

The Mullet may be a democratic phenomenon, but some Mullets simply rise above the rest. A shining beacon in an otherwise mundane universe, Deluxe is what you need when totally over-the-top isn't *quite* enough.

The Cream of the Crop: We know who we are, don't we? Oh yes we do!

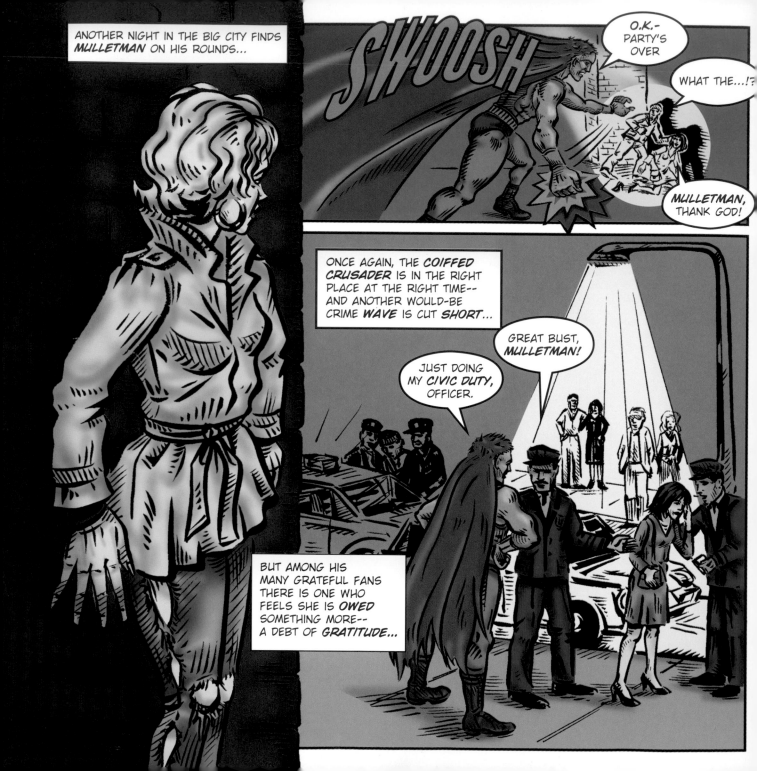

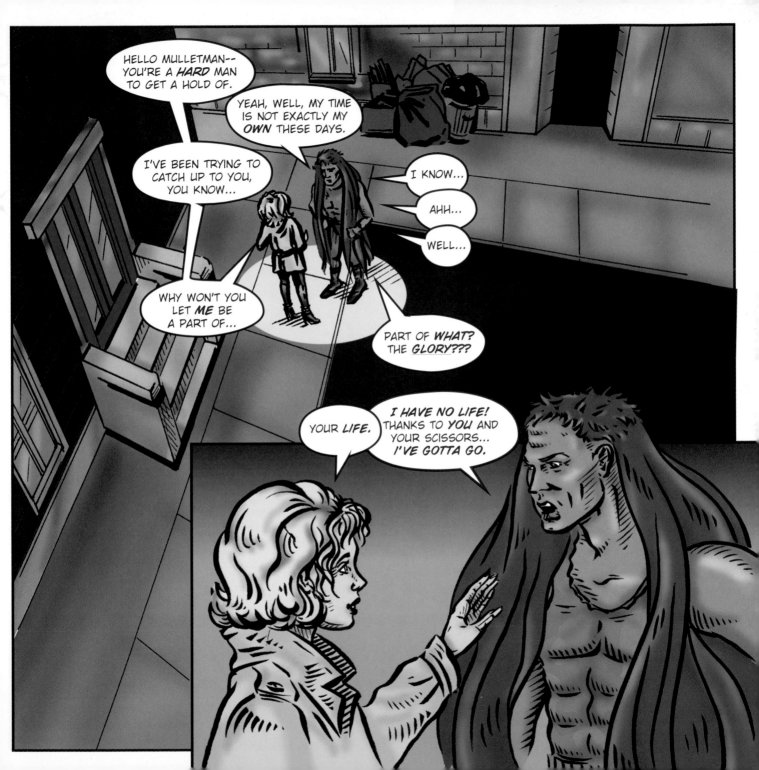

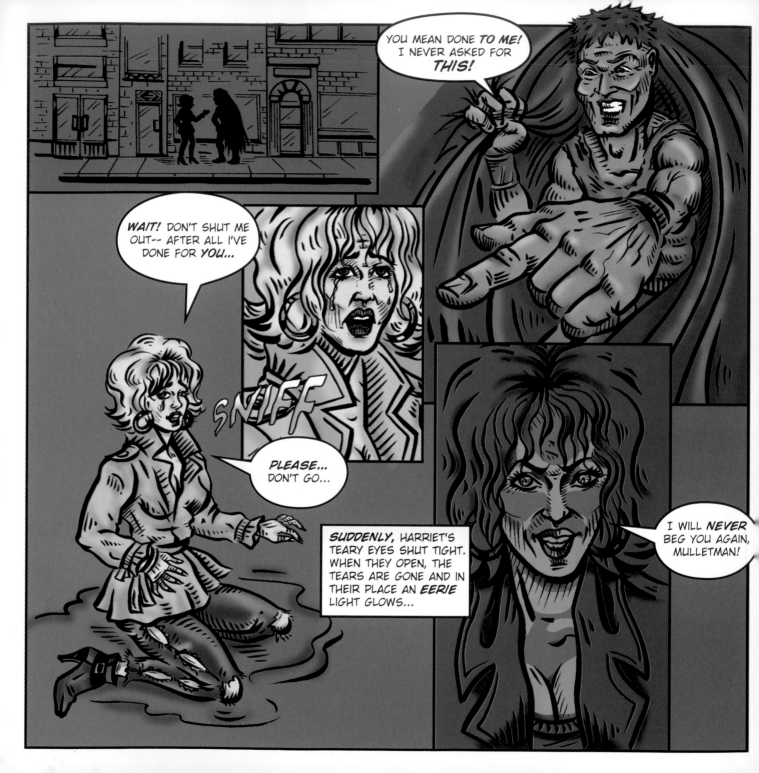

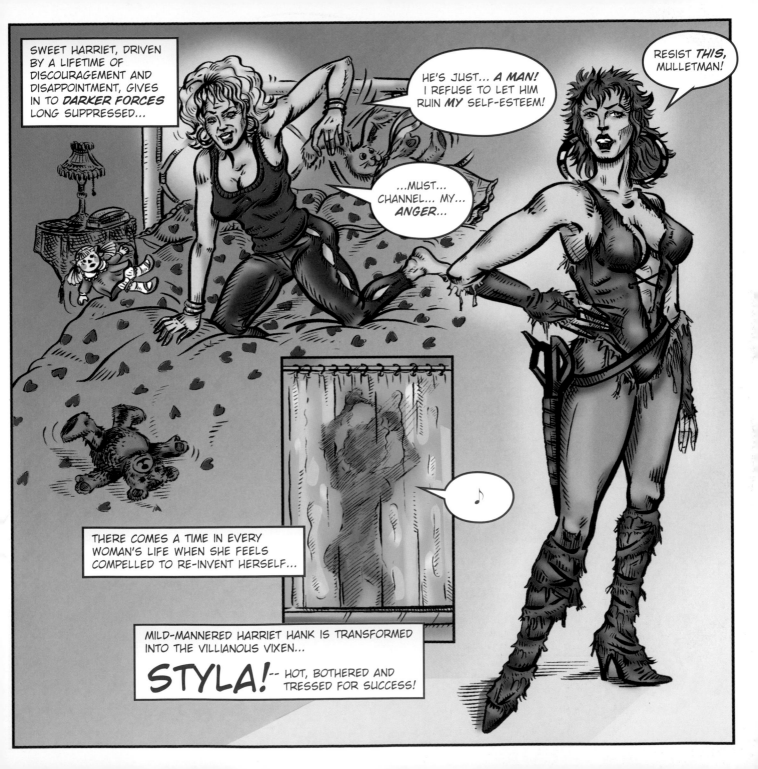

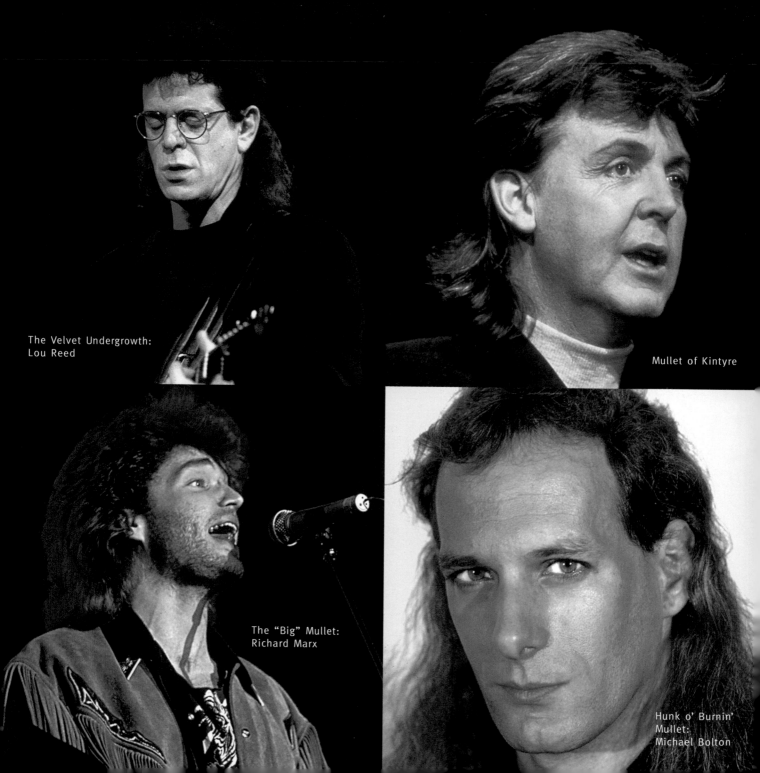

The Velvet Undergrowth:
Lou Reed

Mullet of Kintyre

The "Big" Mullet:
Richard Marx

Hunk o' Burnin'
Mullet:
Michael Bolton

Where would we be without our Celebrity Mullets? The fact that so many famous people have seen fit to go "sho-lo" only confirms the potency and beauteousness of bi-levelism. While the style is quintessentially Everyman (and Woman), stars of screen and field have lent their charisma to the cut from the day David Bowie first metamorphosed into Ziggy Stardust. Just as Samson derived his superhuman strength from his mane, so today's stars would be nothing without their two-tier tresses. *Sans molet*, would Mel Gibson have been half the hero he was in *Lethal Weapon*? Shorn of their Ape Drapes, would wrestlers like Hulk Hogan and Randy Savage have licked so many rivals in the ring? Minus the "Buddhist Rat Tail" Mullet that dangled behind his neck, would soccer maestro Roberto Baggio have been capable of such wizardry? To admit that fame lends the Mullet a certain patina – *a magical radiance* – is not to devalue its intrinsic splendour; it is simply to concede that anything the famous endorse is automatically the greater for their endorsement.

LIKE SAMPSON MY HAIR IS MY POWER AND I WON'T LET NO DAMN DELORIS CUT IT OFF! — LINK D.

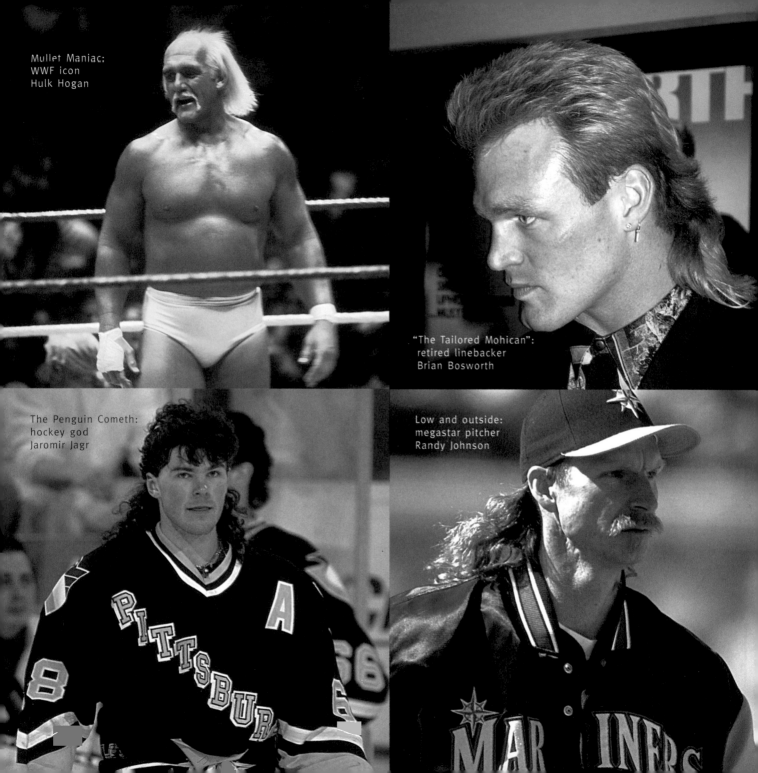

Mullet Maniac:
WWF icon
Hulk Hogan

"The Tailored Mohican":
retired linebacker
Brian Bosworth

The Penguin Cometh:
hockey god
Jaromir Jagr

Low and outside:
megastar pitcher
Randy Johnson

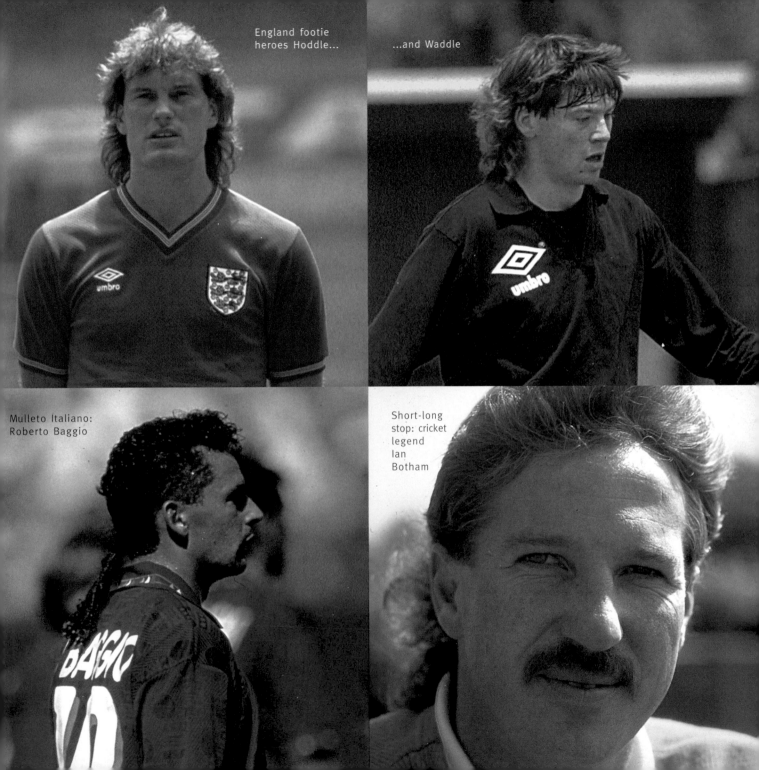

England footie heroes Hoddle...

...and Waddle

Mulleto Italiano: Roberto Baggio

Short-long stop: cricket legend Ian Botham

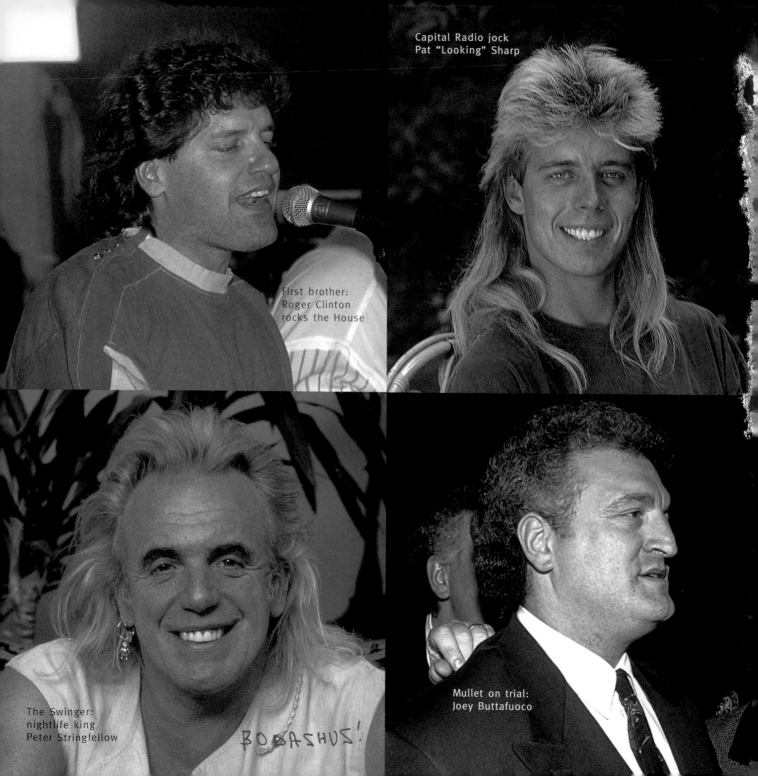

First brother:
Roger Clinton
rocks the House

Capital Radio jock
Pat "Looking" Sharp

The Swinger:
nightlife king
Peter Stringfellow

BODASHUS!

Mullet on trial:
Joey Buttafuoco

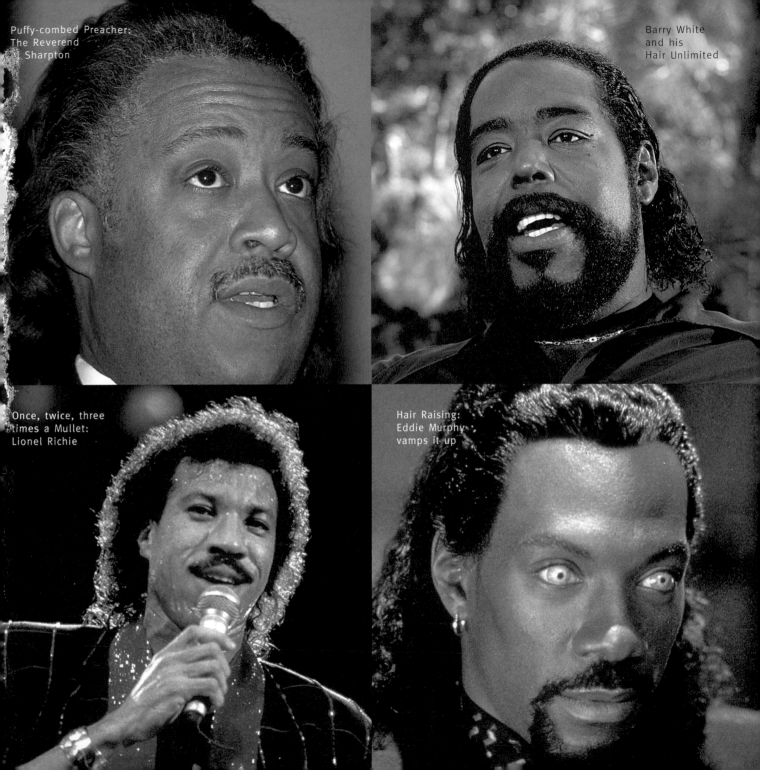

Puffy-combed Preacher:
The Reverend
Sharpton

Barry White
and his
Hair Unlimited

Once, twice, three
times a Mullet:
Lionel Richie

Hair Raising:
Eddie Murphy
vamps it up

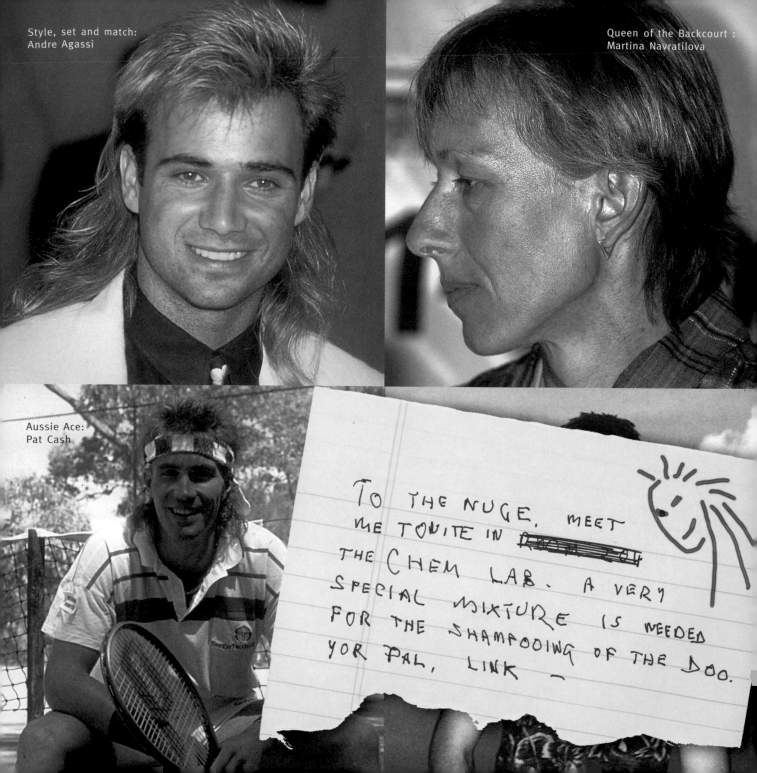

Style, set and match:
Andre Agassi

Queen of the Backcourt :
Martina Navratilova

Aussie Ace:
Pat Cash

TO THE NUGE. MEET
ME TONITE IN ▓▓▓▓▓▓
THE CHEM LAB. A VERY
SPECIAL MIXTURE IS NEEDED
FOR THE SHAMPOOING OF THE DOO.
YOR PAL, LINK —

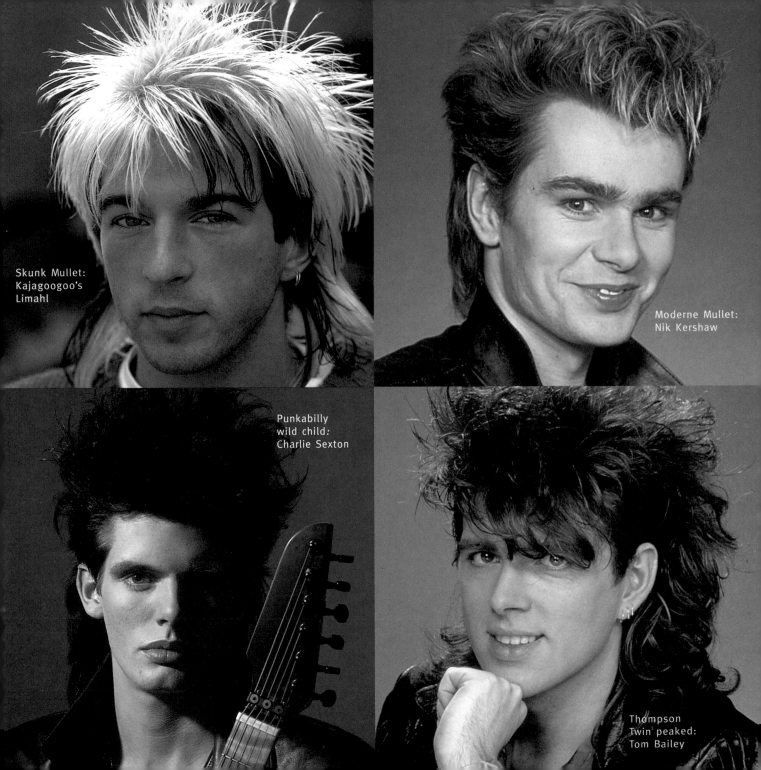

Skunk Mullet: Kajagoogoo's Limahl

Moderne Mullet: Nik Kershaw

Punkabilly wild child: Charlie Sexton

Thompson Twin peaked: Tom Bailey

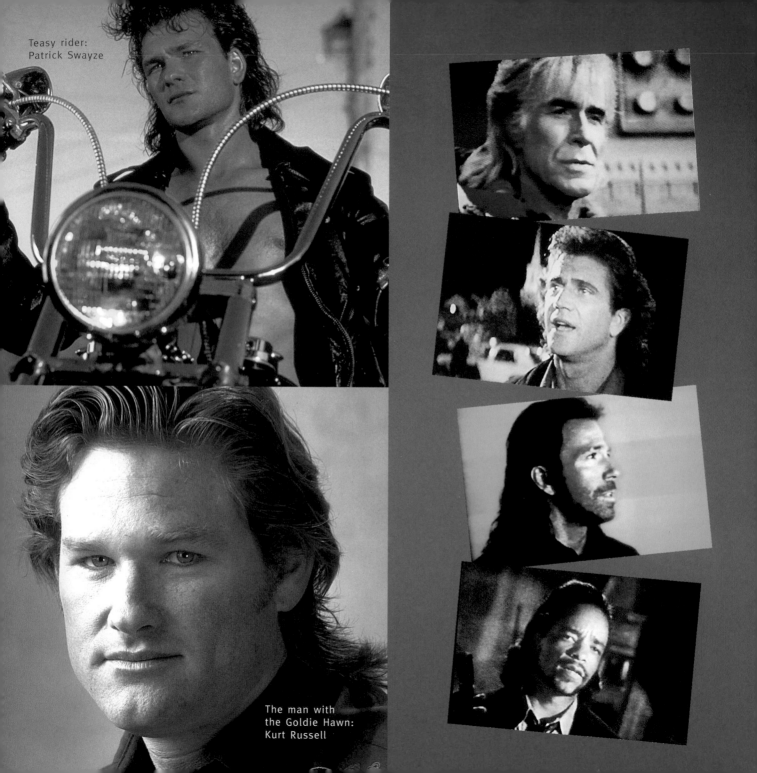

Teasy rider:
Patrick Swayze

The man with
the Goldie Hawn:
Kurt Russell

MULLETS ON FILM

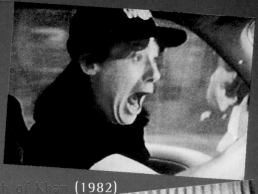

FUTUREMULLET: Ricardo Montalban in *Star Trek II: The Wrath of Khan* (1982)

BUSH MAN: Mel Gibson in *Lethal Weapon 3* (1992)

AVENGING PELT: Chuck Norris in *The Hitman* (1992)

PROCESSED SHO-LO: Ice T in *Trespass* (1992)

WET-LOOK WARRIOR: Jean-Claude Van Damme in *Hard Target* (1993)

MEDIEVAL MANE: Dennis Quaid in *Dragonheart* (1996)

PORNO MOP: Peter Stormare in *The Big Lebowski* (1998)

EIGHTIES DRAPE: Adam Sandler in *The Wedding Singer* (1998)

BI-LEVEL BLACULA: Eddie Murphy in *The Vampire From Brooklyn* (1995)

HEADBANGER: Mike Myers in *Wayne's World 2* (1993)

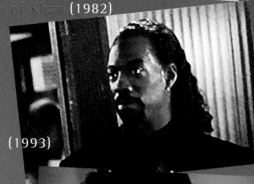

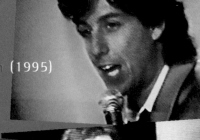

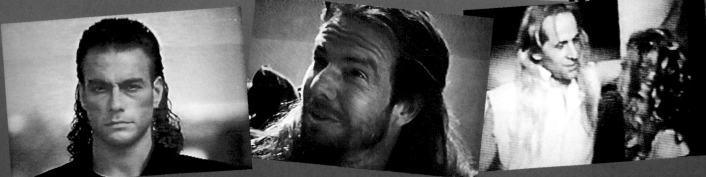

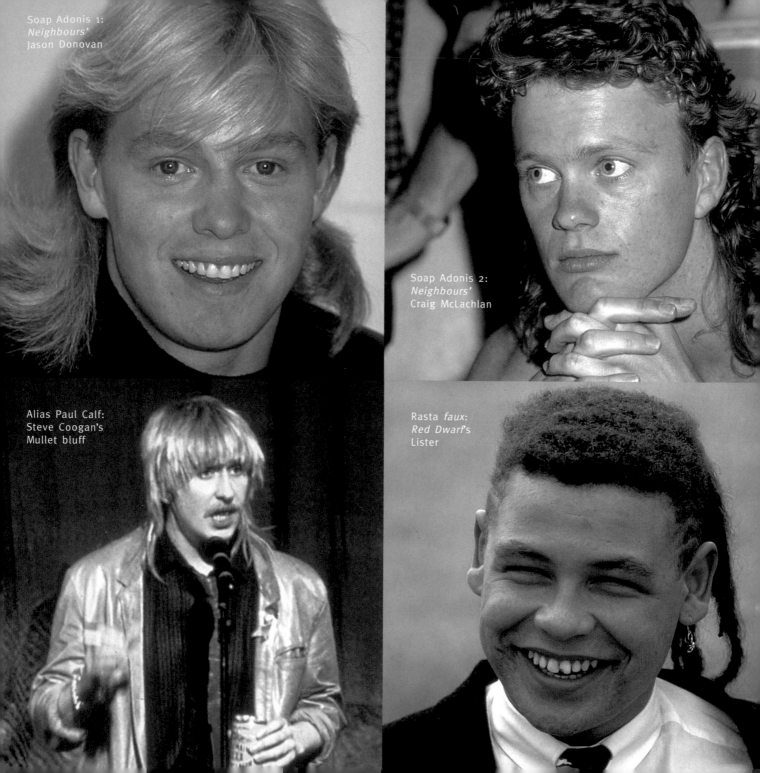

Soap Adonis 1:
Neighbours'
Jason Donovan

Soap Adonis 2:
Neighbours'
Craig McLachlan

Alias Paul Calf:
Steve Coogan's
Mullet bluff

Rasta *faux*:
Red Dwarf's
Lister

Link,
    I know just the thinG.
Mix a littlE of this and a
little of that and poof—
the perFect poo for the doo.
Better living through
chemistry, dude!
                    —THE Nuge

Visit
Seville's
Historic
Flugel
Fountain

Enduring Monument
to Jan Van Flugel,
founder of Seville
*"As long as these waters flow free,
all shall prosper!"*

WILLIAM OF CYRUS

"The Achy Sacred Heart"

A dreamy lad given to wandering through the nearby woods and fields, William in his youth was afflicted with fainting spells. During one such episode he fell and hit his head on a tree stump, dreaming that his entire village had gone bald. The boy awoke and led his people into the woods, beseeching them to daub their pates with pine resin. When an infestation of the dreaded Black Scabie swept through Cyrus, the believers were spared while skeptics suffered the slow and agonizingly itchy loss of their hair. William went on to become a kind and wise leader to his people.

Years later, when the Normans invaded Cyrus, William led a valiant resistance but was eventually captured by the enemy. He was brought to the village square to be publicly humiliated. As his horrified followers looked on, the soldiers cut off the top of his long, flowing hair. Miraculously, he looked even more beautiful, and the villagers promptly ran the discredited Normans out of town.

Though his inspiring story has fallen somewhat into obscurity over the centuries, William remains to many the beloved protector of souls in danger of sudden hair loss.

GLORIA IN PELLUM EST

Behold, for glorious is his hair.

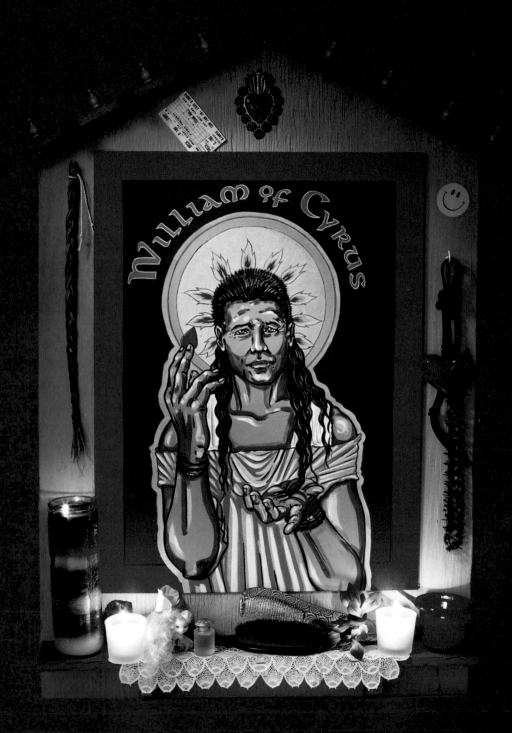

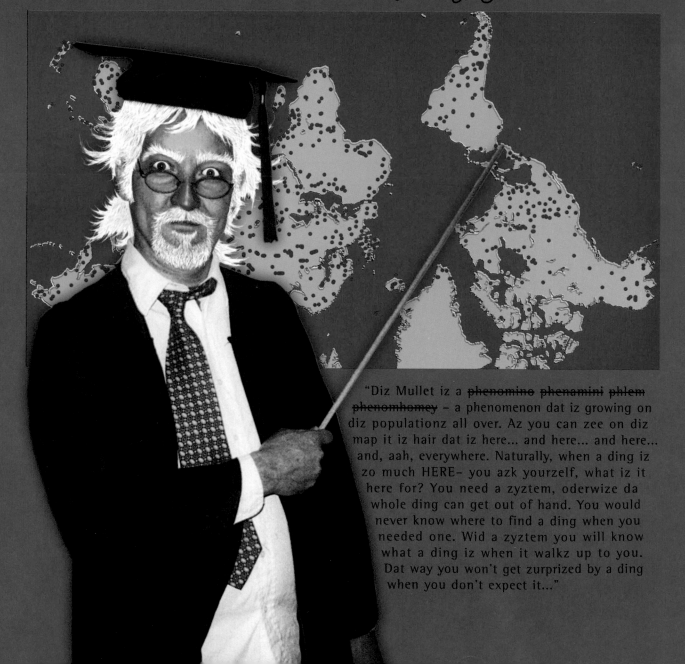

And Now A Word From Prof. Wyngarde Floote...

"Diz Mullet iz a ~~phenomino phenamini phlem phenomhomey~~ – a phenomenon dat iz growing on diz populationz all over. Az you can zee on diz map it iz hair dat iz here... and here... and here... and, aah, everywhere. Naturally, when a ding iz zo much HERE– you azk yourzelf, what iz it here for? You need a zyztem, oderwize da whole ding can get out of hand. You would never know where to find a ding when you needed one. Wid a zyztem you will know what a ding iz when it walkz up to you. Dat way you won't get zurprized by a ding when you don't expect it..."

THE MULLET-WATCHER'S FIELD GUIDE

PROFESSOR WYNGARDE FLOOTE'S PATENTED SYSTEM FOR THE GLOBAL CLASSIFYING OF MULLET VARIETIES, BASED UPON DR. HERBERT BARBEL'S FAMOUS "ORNITHOLOGICAL-ANALOGOUS METHOD" OF 1932.

THRASHERS
THE FLAMING BUSTARD
THE PUFFY-COMBED WAGTAIL
THE TUFTED CONUNDRUM
THE BOOBY
THE FURIOUS BOTTOMSCRATCHER

PECKERS
THE MORNING WOOD
THE DANGLING DICKYBIRD
THE WATTLED LOTHARIO
THE UNCOMMON SHAFTER
THE RED-FACED SHAME-SPIRALLER

DIPPERS
THE TYRANT FLYCATCHER
THE HUGE TIT
THE WHISTLING DUCK
THE PLUMED COOT
THE RUMPED BUNTING

FLAPPERS
THE SHERYL CROW
THE PILIATED SAPSUCKER
THE CREEPING MEGAPODE
THE GREATER-BREASTED BALLBUSTER
THE LESSER-BREASTED NUTSQUEEZER

Leslye Babcock-Marsdale

Brilliant, simply brilliant! Not since he published the seminal *Broccoli in the Himalayas*, the culmination of his fifteen-year-long "Punk Anthropology" series, have we heard from one of the purest voices of his or any other generation. Leslye Babcock-Marsdale, legendary for his almost excruciating attention to detail, resurfaces after ten long years with a new exhibition and forthcoming book. Traveling to the four corners of the globe, leaving no stone unturned and no free meal uneaten, Babcock-Marsdale has trained his unique, all-seeing eye on the cultural phenomenon known as the Mullet. In the stunning new series *In Mullet Country*, he dives deeply into the milieu of his subject. Not content to simply make photographs of the hairstyle, he shows us what lurks within the hairstyle, underneath it, *around* it.

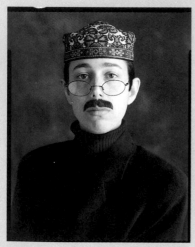

L.B.M.

"I do not 'take' pictures, I 'give' pictures. I am not like these other shutterbugs. Deadlines mean nothing to me. If it takes a week to make one exposure, then that is how long we must wait. You cannot rush genius!"

We couldn't agree more. Nor could we be more pleased to present this advance look at a Mullet masterwork from the self-declared "Mozart of the view camera".

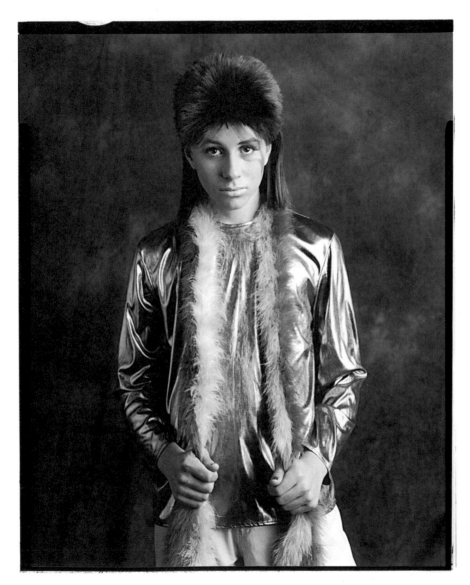

"Ziggy", high school student, Carson City, Nevada 1998

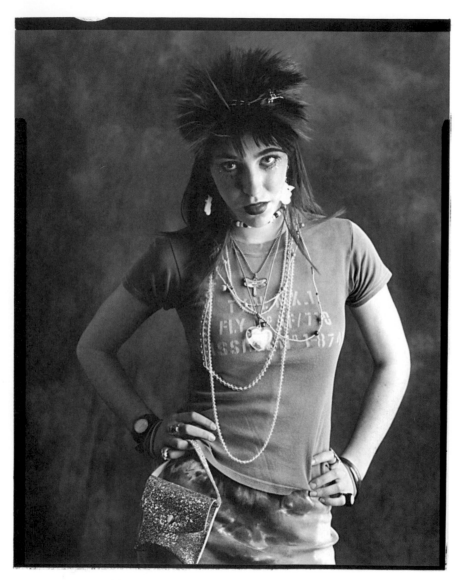

Aspidistra, receptionist, Fond Du Lac, Wisconsin 1997

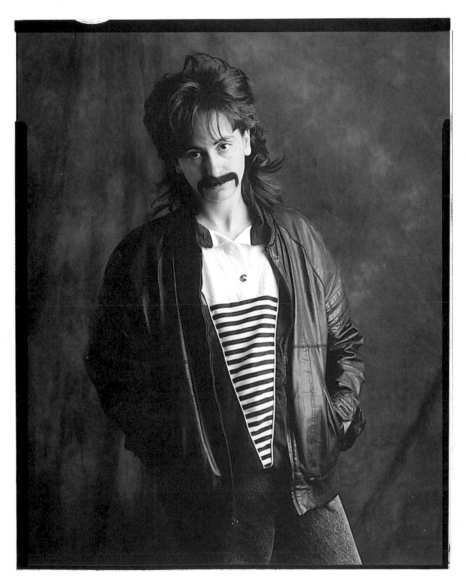

Daryl, scalper, Defiance, Ohio 1998

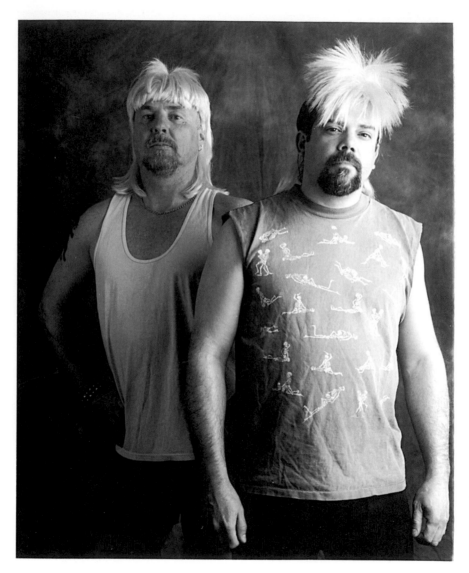

Lothar and "The Hand", amateur wrestlers, Fernandina Beach, Florida 1999

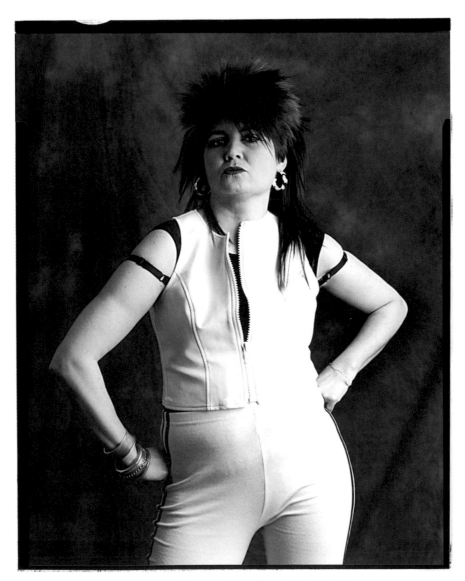

Vera Rivera ("La Niña"), entertainer, Union City, New Jersey 1999

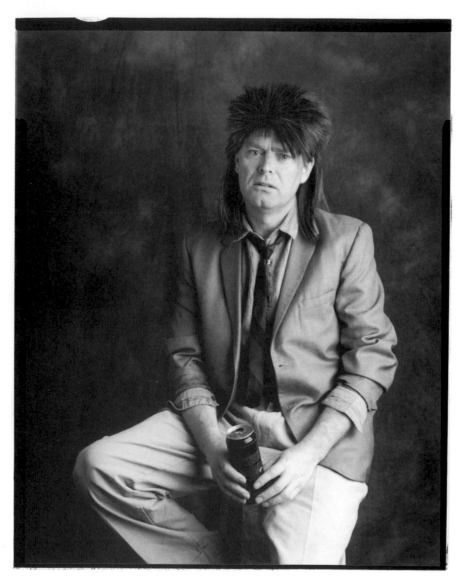

Noel, English bass player, South Pasadena, California 1997

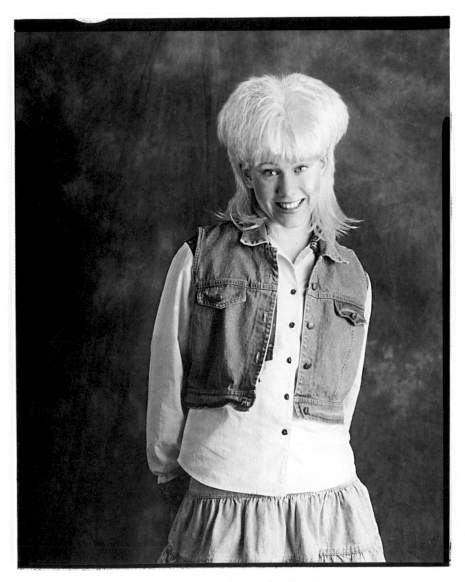

Shanona, LeAnn Rhimes fan, Zunkerville, Texas 1998

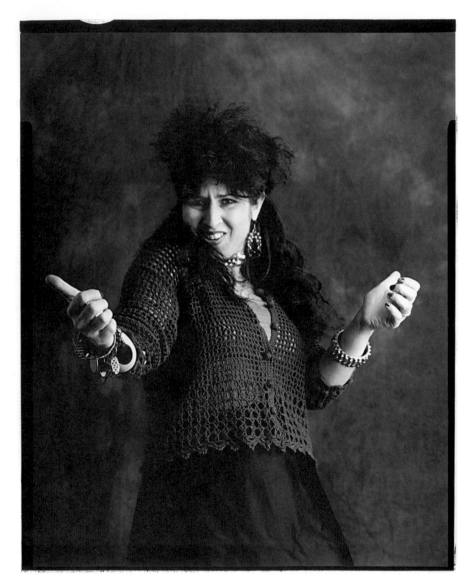

Ronee, party girl, Tempe, Arizona 1998

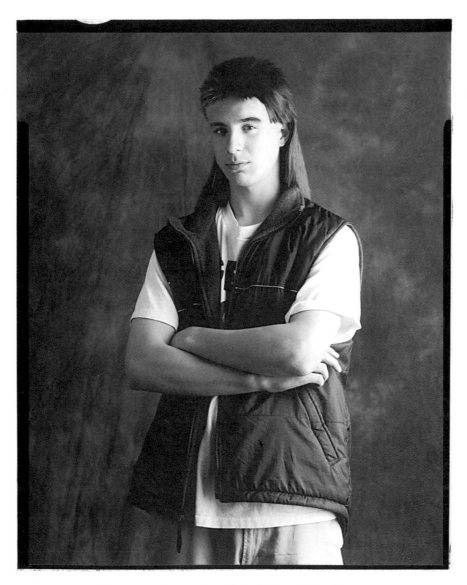

COOL!

Shep, convenience store clerk, Wahoo, Nebraska 1999

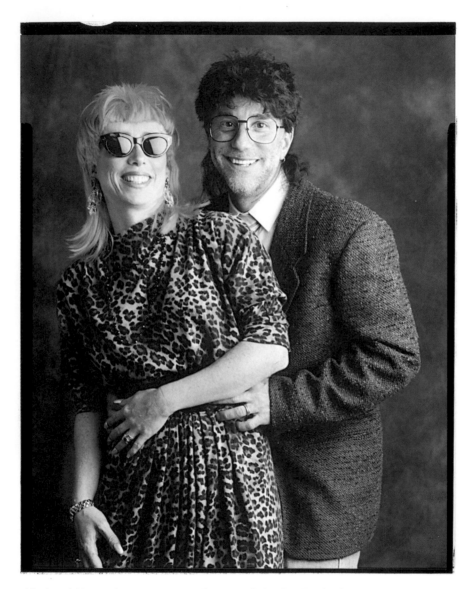

Mitzi and Marty, department store buyer and dentist, Ronkonkoma, New York 1996

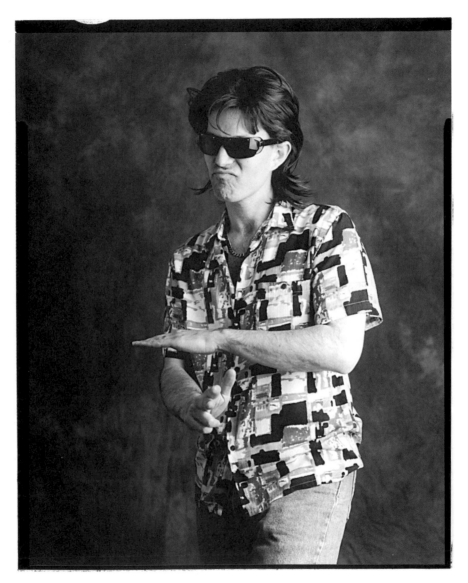

Buff, aspiring film producer, Carbondale, Illinois 1997

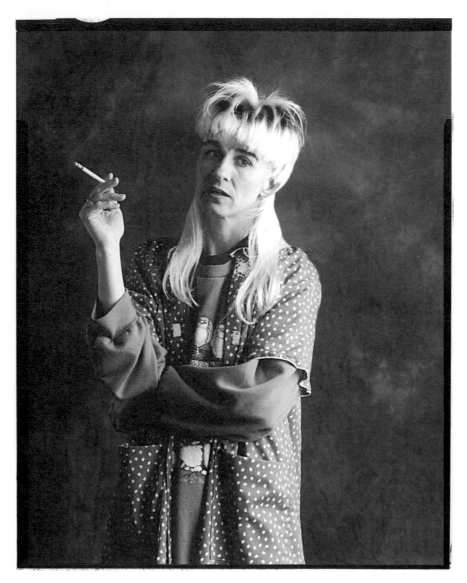

Astrid, housewife and rabbit breeder, Back Gate, Arkansas 1998

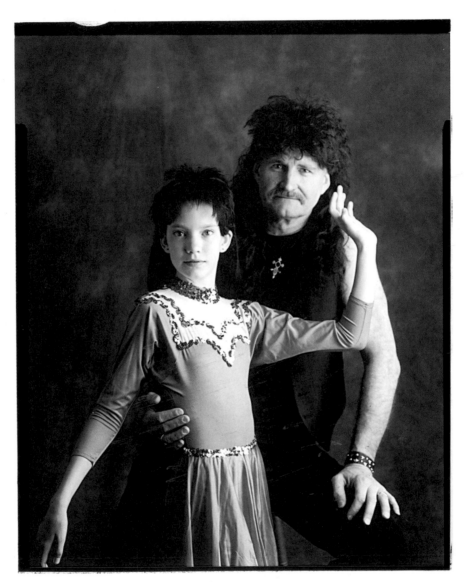

Warthog and Celeste, father and daughter, Moberly, Missouri 1998

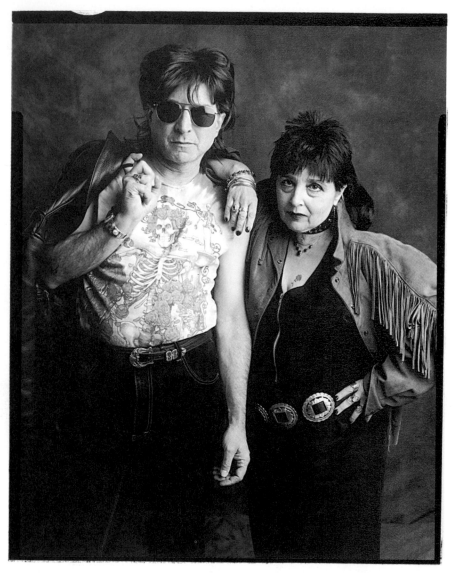

Wolf and Steppen, bikers/taxidermists, Yankton, South Dakota 1999

REAL FASHION IS ON THE INSIDE
AND IT COMES OUT IN YOUR HAIR—
LINK D.

Spotting and Luring your Mullet...

"First you have to find the Mullet! Several hours spent walking and observing the various spots along the shoreline attempting to locate the Mullet will be time well spent. They are normally found very close to shore, mainly at the water's edge. Look for an *agitated or shimmering surface* that stands out from the surrounding area, and by all means WEAR POLAROID GLASSES. Once found, keep in mind that Mullet will often remain in a spot or in a general area for several days, or perhaps even a week or two. Remember too: when they leave, they are heading south."

Ray Bondorew
"The Finer Points of Finding and Imitating Mullet"
http://www.reel-time.com/~sparky/reel-time/feature/travel/R.I./mullet/RBmullet.html

HOW TWO SMALLTOWN PALS
BANDED TOGETHER TO CHAMPION
THE HAIRSTYLE THEY BELIEVED IN

The way Carl Spootz tells it, the first Mullethead in Zenith, Indiana, was a skinny Czechoslovakian dude named Pavel Skurvy.

Skurvy was an exchange student who came to America in 1974 and had a spiritual awakening after watching the film of David Bowie's last "Ziggy Stardust" show. Skurvy was so mesmerized by Bowie's orange Mullet in the film that he marched himself down to his local barber armed with a photo of the singer from *Hit Parader*.

the ng behind

y know, expressing myself," prominent local trash hauler. air 'n stuff, but that was how come then one day I saw ol' Pavel walkin' ria and boy, did *he* stand out!"

tz's barber was rather less understanding than Skurvy's. dy's name was Stokey, and he told me to git or he'd call my

88 *(continued p130)*

MANE MAN

THE MAG FOR THE MODERN MULLETHEAD

$2.95

The Agassi and the Ecstasy
Life Before Brooke

Deep-rooted Desires
Sizzling Tips for Mullet Lovers

Magnificent Mulletmobiles
Finding the right Camaro for you

Stairways to Heaven
Mullet Feng Shui

PLUS!

"I know him, and he does": Inside Geddy Lee

Emerald Dreams: A Pilgrimage to Mullet Bay

Jagr's guide to Lager: Quaffing with Jaromir

Mullet Lovin'

Hot Lips, Hot Hips & Hot Tips!

Hey, Mullet Lovers! Why choose between running your fingers through a lover's silky locks *or* softly passing your open palm over his or her brushy cropped top? When it comes to lovemaking, variety is *definitely* the spice of life! Whether you prefer it silky or shaggy, curly or spiked, the Mullet opens up a world of sensual possibilities...

Two heads are better than one, so if you're lucky enough to be one half of a red-hot Mullet couple, you're already *way* ahead of the game!

Her:

Let's face it, most men are irrationally mad about long hair, whereas most women like to experiment with their look. Now you can have it all. Please your man while pleasuring yourself. The Mullet is the answer to the fulfillment of both your *deep-rooted desires*. For that seductive "bedroom hair" look, sweep the top of your Mullet forward to frame your face. Set the bottom with hot rollers to complete the "tousled" effect. Wear a low-backed dress – your man'll go crazy knowing there's *nothing* between you and your Mullet!

Naughty But Nice:

A little gender-bending can go a *long* way to recharging your love batteries (remember what it did for David Bowie). Not ready for cross-dressing? Try a Mullet swap for a night. We guarantee the sparks will fly!

Him:

Always remember to keep your Mullet squeaky clean and well-groomed if you want to attract the babes. (Don't miss this month's *Care and Feeding* section!) If you're a guy who loves having his ears nibbled we recommend the more radical cropped-back Mullet style. Ask her to whisper sweet nothings and show her you *like* what you hear!

Tips For Mullet Lovers:

Setting the mood:

- Serve your beer in a champagne flute!
- Fill your ashtrays with potpourri – the warm ashes'll bring out the scent! (Cautionary note: watch for those sparks!)
- Dab mouthwash on your pulse points for that "Just-Clean" smell!
- Aroused by chocolate? See this month's Mullet Cuisine snack-cake guide!

Dating Do's & Don'ts

Spotted that perfect Mullethead sitting alone at the bar?

GUYS!

DON'T SAY: "Haven't I seen that haircut somewhere before?"

DO SAY: "Excuse me, aren't you one of the lifeguards on *Baywatch*?"

(*Tip:* Before you approach, discreetly check to see if your fly is open by hooking your thumb over your belt buckle and feeling with your pinky.)

GALS!

DON'T SAY: "Didn't I see you on *America's Most Wanted*?"

DO SAY: "Thank God, a real man at last!"

S O S
(Save our Strands!)

You can't find a barber or stylist who's worthy of cutting your hair. You've flooded us with mail and WE HEAR YOU! So we've put our heads together and come up with this list of 10 outstanding places to go for that perfect cut. (If they're too far afield, don't fret! We'll be featuring further fab salons in upcoming issues.)

1 Repent! Hair Design, Galilee, Texas (USA)

2 Something For the Weekend, Spume-on-Sea (England)

3 Kuntree Kurlz, Burns Flat, Oklahoma (USA)

4 Barberia Jose de Cabezon y Peludo, Santiago (Chile)

5 Billy Splittinghairs' Hair Le Hot, Flagstaff, Arizona (USA)

6 Emporio di Massimo Lunghicorti, Naples (Italy)

7 Ask For Monty's, Queens, New York (USA)

8 Yori Yoi Happy Hair Salon, Osaka (Japan)

9 KrimsKramsKopf Precision Hair, Bremen (Germany)

10 Don't Touch The Outback, Woga Woga (Australia)

SNIPPETS with LARRY PODBILNIAK
Mullethead-at-large

#12 Mullets and "Big Hair": Friends or Foes?

Okay, so *we* all know that "Big Hair" – y'know, the kind worn by heavy metal hairtrees and secretaries from Queens – is way less classy than the Mullet. Yet the two styles have more in common than you might think. For starters, they've both come in for excessive of abuse from trendier-than-thou urban snobs. Snooty Manhattanites, for example, refer to both Mullets and "Big" hairdos as "bridge and tunnel" cuts, as if nobody who lived in the 212 phone zone would be seen dead with either style.

A still deeper connection links Mullets and Big Hair, which is that Camaro-driving Mulletheads simply *adore* women with Big, nay Huge, hair. In his highfalutin' tome *Big Hair: A Journey into the Transformation of Self*, Grant McCracken attributes this to the notion that Big Hair "feels like an act of deference by women to men", but perhaps he's missing the point. Maybe it has more to do with a kind of *hairstyle solidarity* between bi-levellers and "poodle-heads". Think about it.

McCracken also notes an interesting late '80s hybrid of Mullet and Big Hair. Arguing that the "blunt" hairstyle of the '80s female executive was a feminist rejection of bimbo fluffiness, he points instead to a bevelled or "compromise" blunt that mixed toughness with sexiness, capturing a professional look but smuggling in "a certain sensuality or softness in the process". This compromise, McCracken concludes, "let the wearer have her cake and eat it too." Which, when you think about it, is exactly what our beloved Mullet does...

Next month: Mullets and "The Beauty Myth"

Mullet Cuisine

This Month:
Holiday in A Hurry!!

It's Holiday season and you like to *party hearty!* Your head's in the toilet and your folks are due at noon. Don't panic, here's a complete holiday meal you can whip together in about half an hour!

TITANIC TUREEN

You'll need:
One large Iceberg lettuce
Three/four containers prepared onion dip
Family-size bag potato chips

Preparation time: 3 minutes

Cooking time: 0 minutes.

1) Hollow out lettuce and cut bottom to sit flat (see illustration)

2) Fill with dip

3) Serve with chips

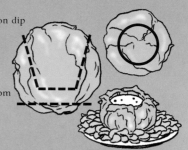

LUNCHEON MEAT DE RESISTANCE

You'll need (allow half a can per serving):
Tinned/canned luncheon meat
Tinned/canned pineapple rings in heavy syrup
One jar maraschino cherries
One bottle barbeque sauce
Cloves (optional)

Preparation time: 8 minutes

Cooking time: 5 minutes

1) Score luncheon meat (see illustration)

2) Brown luncheon meat in heavy frying pan

3) After three minutes, brush meat with barbeque sauce. Continue cooking for two additional minutes. Remove from heat.

4) Place loaf(s) on platter and garnish with lettuce (Titanic leftovers ideal), pineapple rings, cherries and cloves (see illustration)

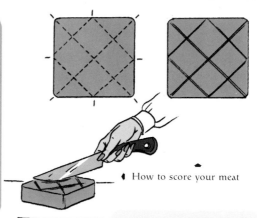

◄ How to score your meat

NO RISK, FOOL-PROOF, EVERY-TIME-A-WINNER CRANBERRY MOULD

You'll need (allow one can per three to four servings):

Tinned/canned Cranberry sauce

Preparation time: 1 minute

Cooking time: 0 minutes

1) Open can, slide onto plate

2) Slice

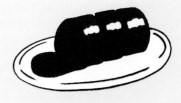

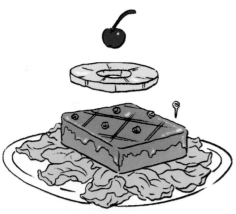

Serving suggestion

And For Dessert...

TWINKIE–MISU

An easy adaptation of the classic Italian delicacy – Mullet style!

We suggest you prepare this first and chill (out!) while enjoying the rest of your meal.

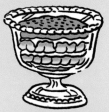

TWINKIE-MISU

You'll need:
1 cup cold, strong, black coffee
1 tin custard or ready-to-eat vanilla pudding
1 can whipped cream or tub of dessert topping
Chocolate sprinkles
4 packages Twinkie Snack Cakes (eight pieces)

Preparation time: Approximately 8 minutes

Refrigeration time: 1 hour

1) Line the bottom of an attractive deep serving dish with cakes
2) Carefully pour coffee over cakes, a little at a time until just moist
3) Spoon on half the custard, spread evenly – repeat for additional layers
5) Top with whipped cream/creme topping & decorate with sprinkles
7) Refrigerate for one hour before serving

Conspicuous Consumer Snack Cake Ratings Guide

Where comfort is concerned, where would we be without our snack cakes? Individually wrapped, available in hundreds of forms, they're irresistible. Ignore the fitness gurus and diet doctors! Why deny yourself childhood's favourite treats when you can have your cake and scoff it too?

Rating:
GOOD/BETTER/BEST

Product type/Description	Brand Name	Product Name	Price Point	Comments	Overall Rating	
I. Chocolate cake sandwich with creme filling	Hostess	Suzy Q's	₵₵₵	More moist and chewy than its counterparts. BUT greasy. Creme is foamy and has synthetic aftertaste. Highest price.	GOOD	
	Drakes	Devil Dog	₵₵	Light, cakey texture. Fluffy, flavourful creme. Most unique chocolate flavour. BUT tendency to dryness. Medium price.	GOOD	
	Little Debbie	Devil Cremes	₵	Cocoa-rich chocolate taste. Light, cakey texture. BUT creme is slightly too sweet. Budget price.	BEST	
II. Creme-filled chocolate cake roll with chocolate icing	Hostess	Ho Ho's	₵₵₵	Good chocolatey taste and texture. BUT creme is foamy and has synthetic aftertaste. Highest-priced in group.	GOOD	
	Drakes	Yodels	₵₵	Great dark-chocolate icing. Generous amount of cake. Fluffy creme. No BUTS about it, this is our favourite! Medium price.	BEST	★ BEST
	Little Debbie	Swiss Rolls	₵	Great for the price. Good cake texture. Fluffy creme. BUT slightly bland icing. Budget price.	GOOD	
III. Iced Devil's-food cupcake with creme center	Hostess	Hostess Cupcake	₵₵₵	Cake texture and taste acceptable. Pleasing decorative motif. BUT frosting taste and texture below par. Creme is foamy and with synthetic aftertaste. Highest price.	GOOD	
	Drakes	Ring Dings	₵₵	Great dark chocolate icing. Moist cake. Iced all over. Fluffy creme. BUT lacks traditional cupcake form. Medium price.	BEST	
	Little Debbie	Chocolate Cupcakes	₵	Exceptional hexagonal shape. Iced top and sides. Rich devils'-food cake. Fluffy creme. Pleasing decorative motif. BUT icing is waxy. Budget price.	GOOD	

· CARE AND FEEDING

Allowing for a wide diversity of hair types and personal style preferences, it's always important to put your best hair forward. To this end, we offer the following easy-care tips:

❶ WASHING

If you're perplexed about how often to wash your two-tiered hair, bear this in mind: short hair may appear oilier than longer locks, thereby requiring more frequent washing. The trick is to shampoo the top tier more often than the lower level. Using a small amount of mild shampoo, work into short hair, then rinse. Long hair should only be washed when it looks or feels dirty. We suggest no more than twice a week.

❷ CONDITIONING

For short hair, "less is more" when it comes to conditioning. As long as you keep the top cropped, try conditioning the bottom only with a "detangling" product whenever you shampoo. If your Mullet is extra long, you may also need to apply a leave-in conditioner on the tips from time to time. (N.B. For maximum sheen, treat your tresses to a hot oil treatment once a month!)

❸ STYLING

Let's face it, there's no haircut like the Mullet for "shear" versatility. Remember these cardinal rules:

natural bristle brushes are kinder to your hair (fewer of those unsightly split ends), and overuse of heat appliances such as dryers or curling tongs can cause pemanent hair damage. Styling options are endless– but we've made a few suggestions below. Try mixing and matching for good times galore!

–THE SHORT HAIRS

❶ Spiky: Work a large dab of "Super-Hold" gel or mousse into hair. Use fingertips to push hair up on end.

❷ Curly: If long enough, set wet, shorter hair on small to medium rollers (use plenty of styling gel). When completely dry, carefully remove rollers. For that fetching baby-doll look, leave curls as they are or gently brush them out for a softer, more sophisticated look.

❸ Smooth: Not for the faint-hearted. To release the sleek jungle-cat in you, apply plenty of styling gel to wet hair and comb straight back.

–THE LONG HAIRS

❶ Plaited: Here's an unusual "twist" for your Mullet.

You don't need to travel the globe to experience a world of style. Let the plait be your passport to new horizons. *Heap big bored?* Divide long hair in two and pull forward. Plait each half, fasten three inches from bottom. *Heidi envy?* Divide long hair. Pull each half out to side while plaiting. Fasten as close to bottom as possible. Clip end of each braid behind ears. Decorate with brightly-coloured ribbon if desired. *Rather be Lyin' with Zion?* Separate hair into many small sections. Plait each section individually. Add an attractive bead to each end!

❷ Tied Up: Pull back long hair into a ponytail if you want to "hi-light" the top of your mop. For formal occasions, gather the ponytail under and pin into a chignon at the nape of the neck. Use spray to hold.

❸ Loose: Whether you have cascading curls or a long flowing Mane™, it always feels good to let your hair down. If you've followed our washing and conditioning tips, you can't go wrong!

#1 With A Mullet!

Our monthly Mullet Rock parade, courtesy of Mervyn's Disc-o-Rama, Pontefract, Wales

Tracks

THIS MONTH (LAST MONTH)

1 (1) **Mullet Head** Beastie Boys (1994)

2 (6) **Head Games** Foreigner (1979)

3 (5) **Long Tall Shorty** Tommy Tucker (1964)

4 (3) **Almost Cut My Hair** Crosby, Stills, Nash & Young (1970)

5 (2) **Get Behind Me** Scott Walker (1969)

6 (21) **Standing On The Top** The Temptations featuring Rick James (1982)

7 (14) **Back When My Hair Was Short** Gunhill Road (1973)

8 (4) **Oops Upside Your Head** The Gap Band (1980)

9 (13) **The First Cut Is The Deepest** P.P. Arnold (1967)

10 (7) **Going Out The Back Way** Johnny Hodges (1944)

Albums

THIS MONTH (LAST MONTH)

1 (4) *The Prime Of Shorty Long* Shorty Long (1969)

2 (20) *Drop That Bottom* L'Trimm (1989)

3 (1) *No More Lookin' Over My Shoulder* Travis Tritt (1998)

4 (7) *Cuts Both Ways* Gloria Estefan (1989)

5 (5) *Permanent Waves* Rush (1980)

6 (6) *The Final Cut* Pink Floyd (1983)

7 (11) *Repeat Offender* Richard Marx (1989)

8 (17) *Heat Treatment* Graham Parker & The Rumour (1976)

9 (10) *Hairway To Steven* Butthole Surfers (1988)

10 (2) *Check Your Head* Beastie Boys (1992)

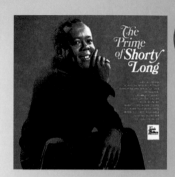

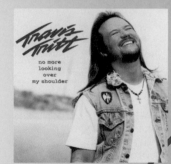

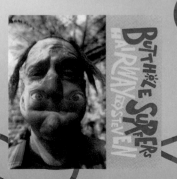

MULLETIN BOARD

Gentlepeople,

I feel I need to share my story with you.

Hair has always been a big thing in my life. Lou, my ex-life partner, and I met at the original Woodstock festival. Among the thousands of free spirits, we found each other and spent the weekend in bliss (our son Ganesh was conceived there). In fact, we never left!!

Even in Woodstock, being a family of longhairs wasn't always easy. Jobhunting proved difficult for Lou and the schools weren't so tolerant then of little boys with shoulder-length hair (some things at least have changed for the better – *right on!*). We persevered, though, and settled into a mellow life with a supportive and loving network of friends.

Imagine how flipped out we were when Ganny came home one day (Oct. 31, 1984 – I'll never forget) with the top of his beautiful hair *cut off!* After all the *sacrifices* and *abuse* we had endured as a family (the horrible jokes that still sting after all these years, the broken ties with relatives), it felt like he was rejecting *our values!*

No amount of family counseling or chamomile could calm my spirit those first few days. Thank the Great Spirit, my friends intervened and guided me through a 24-hour session of meditation and prayer. I came to totally accept that my boy was simply struggling to *define himself* as *we* had years before. We found a new peace as a family.

Just as we reached this plateau, Ganny cut off his Mullet (of course I didn't know it had a name then). This wasn't as difficult a transition (to my surprise, whenever I looked over and saw his newly shaved head, I think I secretly missed his Mullet a little). Time passed, my kids grew up and are (pretty much) on their own. Lou found a younger life partner last year (*no* judgements – men deal with the ageing process differently.)

Two months ago I attended my regular Thursday evening womyn's drumming circle (Sisters of the Change *rule!*) when in walked a very intense new member. Something about her look was vaguely familiar... *She had a Mullet!* It had been years since I'd seen one and, suffice it to say, I experienced a very profound karmic reaction.

To make a "long" story "short" (ha ha!) Frida's hairstyle has caught on with some of the sisters and I am now a complete convert! My Mullet has given me a new lease on life. It took years off my appearance and has (literally) lifted a weight off my crown chakra just as it's coming into its fullness. Life has never been better!!!

When I heard about your magazine, it was like a sign from the universe. I hope you will share this offering with your readers.

Yours in peace and pride,
Sapphlower LeVine
Woodstock, N.Y.

Dear Sapph,

Your letter was *so* moving – there's not a dry eye in the house. Thanks for spreading the good word!

MB

Dear Mulletin Board,

I've been a Mullet wearer for years now and it's always fit my rebel lifestyle.

After years of just scraping by, I'd finally had it (actually, my wife did) and decided to try and get a regular gig. A friend suggested I hide my Mullet to improve my chances of getting hired.

I tied back and tucked in my hair, swallowed my pride and went for my first interview. It worked! Now I'm supposed to start training at the bank on Monday and I'm a little confused. Does this mean I can *never* wear my Mullet down? Should I show it up front so they get used to it right away?

Joining the Ranks

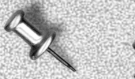

Dear Joining,

The Mullet has been unfairly characterized as the haircut of the marginally employed for way too long. Of course we know, don't we, that there are Mullets in all walks of life, on every rung of the social ladder. But your friend has a point – there are some businesses in which a more conservative look is preferred.

Since you were hired as much on the basis of your appearance as on your skill and life experience, you'd be wise to take it slow at first. Keep your hair tied up and hidden for, say, the first six months. We know what a sacrifice this is, but ensuring your success should be priority number one right now.

Once your co-workers and bosses have gotten to know you, there will no doubt be an opportunity to "let your hair down" at a company softball game or picnic, off-hours.

By then they'll *know* what an asset you are!

MB

P.S. For further support, check out your local chapter of the Retired Mulleted Executives' Network. A great group of guys!

Dear Mulletin Board,

I have this incredibly curly hair that gets frizzy and out of control in humid weather, right? Anyway, I'm going on vacation to the Caribbean in 2 weeks and I'd *love* to take the plunge and get a Mullet before I go (I've thought about it for almost a year now.) Problem is, I'm afraid I'll look like one of those really *big* poodles the first time I'm caught in a tropical rainstorm. Help!

Frizzy in Frisco

Dear Frizzy,

Don't fret – the possibilities are endless! Though your concern is understandable, we feel it shows you've had limited experience in the world of Mullet style. There are Mullets in all shapes and sizes and for all hair types. With the proper care and conditioning we're confident you can always look your best, regardless of the weather. Of course you should always consult a professional before such a drastic change.

Last but not least, with such an abundance of hair (lucky devil!), perhaps a more "ethnic" look would work for you. You *could* postpone your cut and use this as a "research" trip. Try one of those braided island "dos" while you're tanning on the beach and be sure to take lots of photos to show your stylist when you get home.

Either way, you can't lose. We're *certain* your new "natty dreads" will bring you lots of "good vibes."

MB

Dear Mulletin Board,

I recently met a girl I really dig at a bar and, well, one thing led to another. I guess she must have been pretty smashed or something, because the next morning she looked kind of horrified. Since I've been told I'm pretty good-looking, I can only think it must have been my Mullet. (It's the first time this ever happened to me.)

I've tried calling her but she won't answer my calls. She was so *hot* I know I've *got* to see her again. I'm even thinking of cutting my hair. What should I do?

Desperate in Duluth

Dear Desperate,

What are you, crazy? Get a grip, man! We know how hard it can be to find the right woman (believe me), but your Mullet is more than a hank of hair. Do we need to remind you that it is a symbol of your very *spirit??* If she digs *you*, she'll dig your Mullet. If she doesn't, good riddance to bad rubbish. That you're even *considering* a cut is alarming – let her go, *before* you do anything rash.

Hold on, bro. Ms. Right is out there, waiting for you!

MB

PS. When was the last time you changed your sheets?

✳

Mullet Living

SO, YOU'VE GOT THE HAIRCUT, NOW WHAT?

Good morning all you out there in *Mulletland*. It's time to wake up and smell the hairgel! There's a style wave sweeping across the continents– a little thing I like to call **"Mullet Living"**. You've got the cut and you're thinking, "Where's the party?" But there's a whole lot more to this than Friday or Saturday night. Oh, yes, Mr. Wednesday afternoon! It's more than a haircut, it's a lifestyle!

STAIRWAY TO HEAVEN: TURN THAT WINDOWLESS BASEMENT ROOM INTO YOUR PSYCHEDELIC DREAM DEN!

What you'll need:
- One windowless room (check downstairs)
- One awesome stereo with *major* speakers (bigger always better)
- Lots of old rugs (color doesn't matter, you can mix and match)
- One lava lamp
- Black light bulbs
- Posters (day-glo)
- Black paint
- Aluminum foil
- Candles, candles, candles…

First, paint *everything* with the black paint. Really lather it up. Getting rid of all ordinary color is a must. Let the paint dry and pin some posters on the wall. Choose your posters carefully. What are your friends into? Nothing breaks up a chilled-out get-together like a heated argument. (You know, Heavy Metal vs Death Metal vs Speed Metal…)

Accoustics are vitally important. Glueing some egg cartons on the back of the door will keep *your* sound in and *their* sound out.

Cover the ceiling with the foil for a (cheaper than) mirror effect. The foil will bounce light around in a trippy sort of way.

Which brings us to the question:

IS BLACK LIGHT ALWAYS APPROPRIATE?

One word: *Yes!* Black light is the ultimate in psycho-pharmacological lighting. It makes your teeth glow in a real attractive way. Mount black lights high on the wall to take advantage of the effect on day-glo posters which actually light up even though it's dark. (Why <u>do</u> they call it *day*-glo?)

with Lance Stewart

So now you say, "Where do I sit?"

One word: fluffy pillows! Loads of them everywhere. Oh, forgot the rugs– pick up the pillows for a minute and put down those rugs I told you to get. Doesn't matter where you put them as long as you've got a bunch. Overlap them everywhere– have fun with it! Ask yourself: if I fall down, will it hurt? If the answer's yes, you haven't gone far enough. Now make with the pillows.

Cool idea: Wrap your candles with foil, make sure the foil extends higher than the candle. Poke holes in the foil to let stars of light through. The effect will be psycherrific! (P.S. You cannot have too many candles. They are considered very *romantic*, and you know what that can mean.)

Cool idea II: Recycling begins at home... leftover beer cans make beautiful and affordable wall sconces. Just cut in half the long way. Cut 'em in half the short way to make a perfect ashtray or candy dish. Be creative, but be sure to bend the sharp part over so you don't get cut.

O.K. You're about ready. Be sure to dress for excess. Fire up the black lights and the lava lamp. Light the incense. Put some Zep on the box and turn it *way* up. I'll see you when you get back. (*If you do!*)

Peace, love and don't touch the back,

Lance

Coming next month:
YOUR VAN AS PLUSH CHAMBER
Turn that wreck into a hot place to crash!
THE MULLET MENU Your late nite diner favorites– make 'em at home in less time than it takes to sing "Paradise City".

In this issue:

Look for my column *What's Hot/What's Rot* for a complete rundown on **Mullet Feng Shui.** Which is the Chinese way of making sure your pad is a place where you can get lucky. Remember, the Chinese have been wearing those Mullet things down their backs for, like, *thousands* of years! So they must know a thing or two.

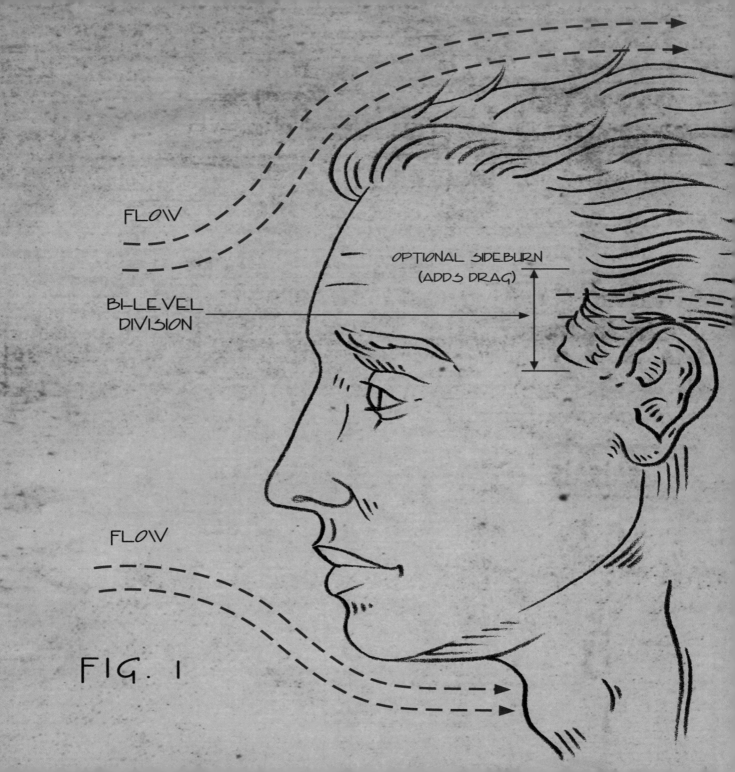

FLOW

BI-LEVEL
DIVISION

OPTIONAL SIDEBURN
(ADDS DRAG)

FLOW

FIG. 1

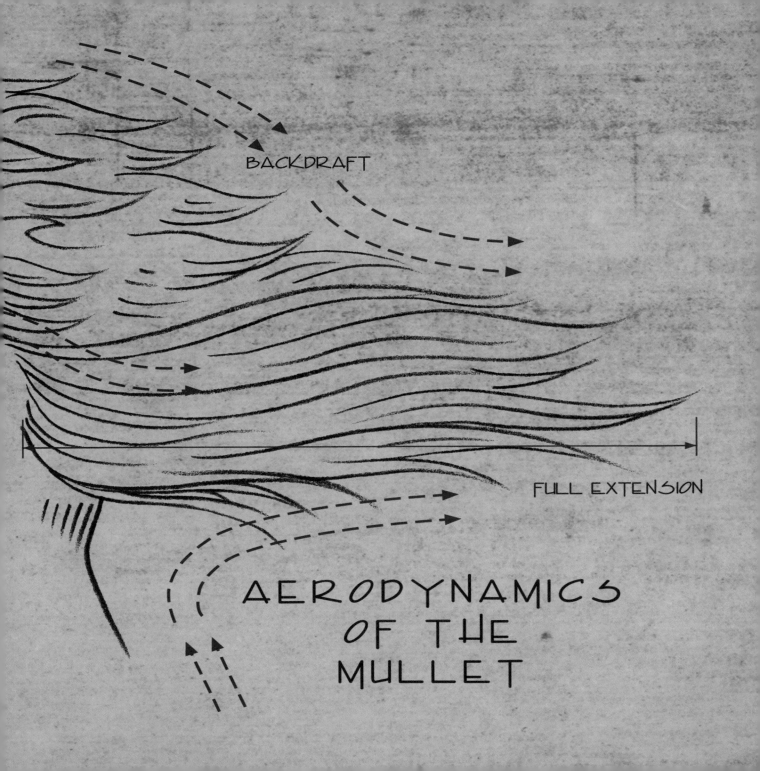

BACKDRAFT

FULL EXTENSION

AERODYNAMICS
OF THE
MULLET

Mulletalia!

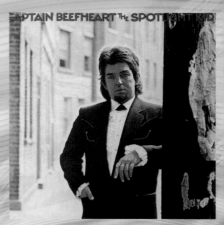

THE LAND MULLET

(Egernia Major) Also known as: a major skink. A shy and swift moving lizard; scuttles away when confronted.
Likes: sunsets and long walks on the beach.

Dental hygienist Mary Lou Biddles describes a recent encounter: "I thought he was interesting – we met at a club. He said he was from Australia. I loved the accent. But then he didn't even call! He really is a <u>major</u> skink!"

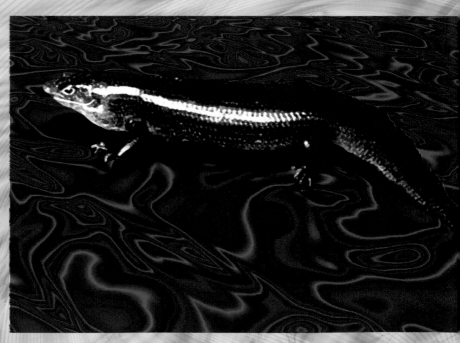

EGERNIA MAJOR, stepping out at The Psychedelic Iguana Club

The Mullet National Anthem
"MORE THAN A HAIRCUT"

(To be rendered to the tune of Boston's "More Than A Feeling",
as interpreted on Ye Olde Space Bande: The Moog Cookbook Plays Classic
Rock Hits, Restless Records, 1997)

Verse
I woke up this morning and no one was there
Walked up to the mirror, I looked so fine
I lost myself in a loving stare
I touched my hair and the world was mine

Chorus
It's more than a haircut (More than a haircut)
When I think of the styles that I used to wear
I feel it in my gut (Feel it in my gut)
Have you ever seen lovelier hair?
I've never ever seen lovelier hair...

When night time comes and I'm on the town
The music is right and I'm feeling good
I think of those times when my hair let me down
But now it's looking the way that it should

It's more than a haircut (More than a haircut)
When I think of the styles I used to wear
I feel it in my gut (Feel it in my gut)
Have you ever seen lovelier hair?
I've never ever seen lovelier hair...

(lather, rinse, repeat)

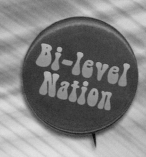

Smells like...

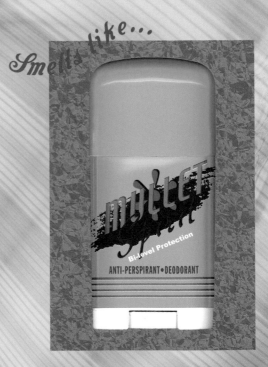

ANTI-PERSPIRANT • DEODORANT

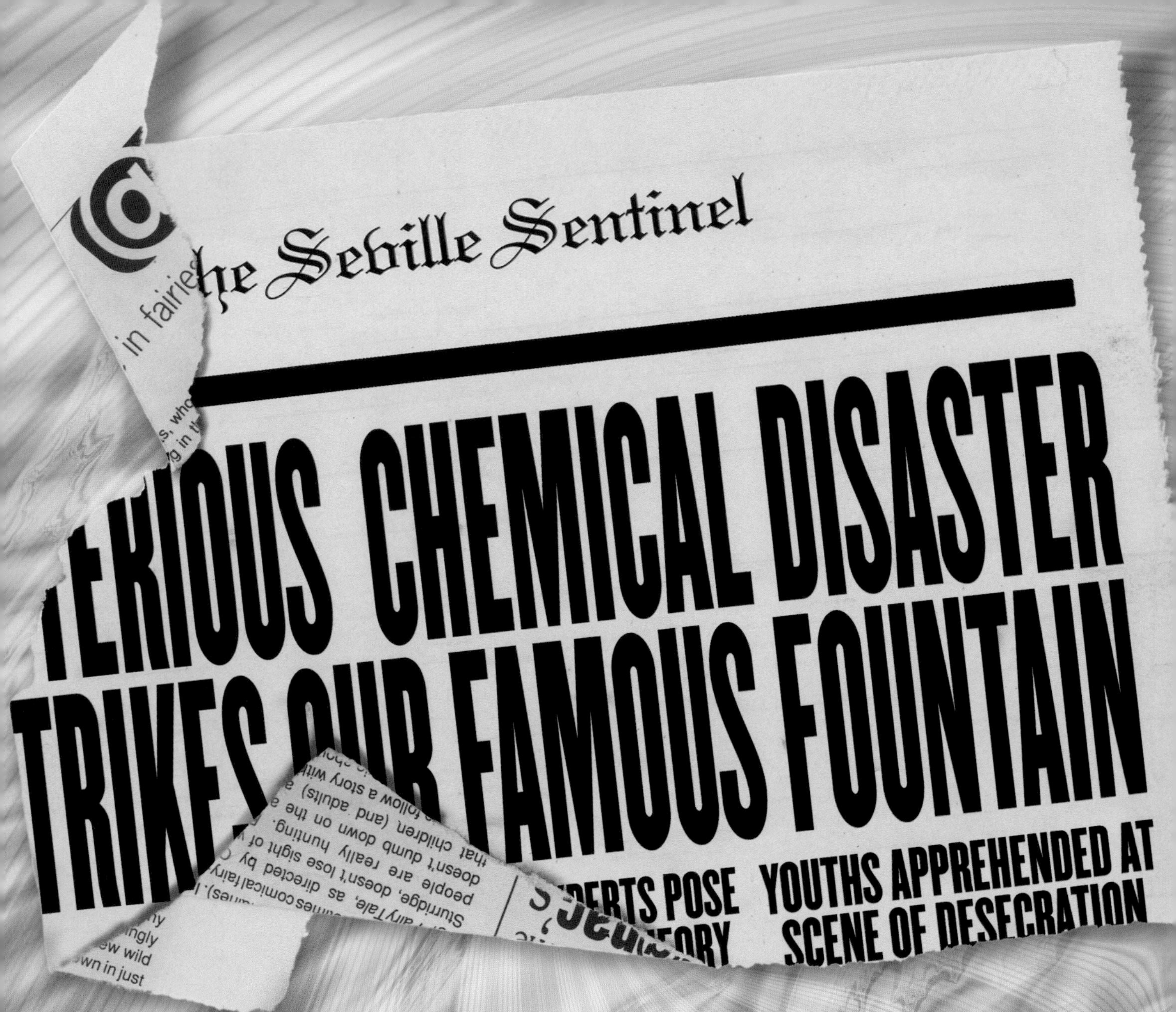

... in fairie

The Seville Sentinel

...TERIOUS CHEMICAL DISASTER
...TRIKES OUR FAMOUS FOUNTAIN

...at children (and adults) a
...doesn't dumb down on the
...people are really hunting,
...Sturbridge, doesn't lose sight of
...fairytale, as directed by
...comes comical fairy

...ingly
...ew wild
...own in just

...ERTS POSE
...HEORY

YOUTHS APPREHENDED AT
SCENE OF DESECRATION

strands

A Quarterly Bulletin of the American Trichological Institute
University of South Northeastern Kansas at Rancid

Vol III, No. 7

Special Issue: Decoding the Mullet

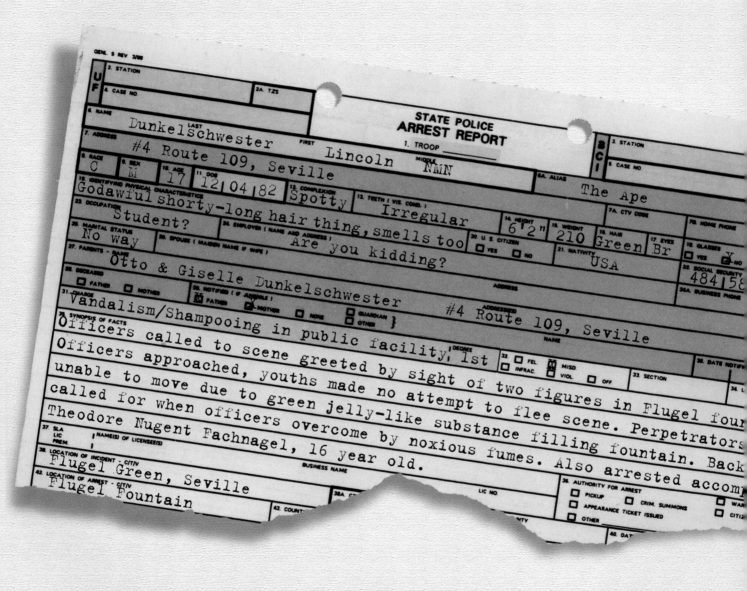

STATE POLICE
ARREST REPORT

GENL S REV 3/80

UF	2. STATION		
	4. CASE NO.	2A. TZS	

1. TROOP _____

BCI	3. STATION
	5 CASE NO

6. NAME LAST Dunkelschwester FIRST Lincoln MIDDLE NMN

6A. ALIAS The Ape

7. ADDRESS #4 Route 109, Seville

8. RACE C 9. SEX M 10. AGE 17 11. DOB 12 04 82 12 COMPLEXION Spotty

13. TEETH (VIS. COND.) Irregular 14. HEIGHT 6'2" 15. WEIGHT 210 16. HAIR Green 17 EYES Br

7A. CTY CODE 7B. HOME PHONE 18. GLASSES ☐ YES ☒ NO

19. IDENTIFYING PHYSICAL CHARACTERISTICS Godawful shorty-long hair thing, smells too

20. U. S. CITIZEN ☐ YES ☐ NO 21. NATIVITY USA

22. OCCUPATION Student?

23A. MARITAL STATUS No way

23. EMPLOYER (NAME AND ADDRESS) Are you kidding?

22. SOCIAL SECURITY 484 58

26. SPOUSE (MAIDEN NAME IF WIFE)

24A. BUSINESS PHONE

27. PARENTS - NAME Otto & Giselle Dunkelschwester

ADDRESS #4 Route 109, Seville

28. DECEASED ☐ FATHER ☐ MOTHER 30. NOTIFIED (IF JUVENILE) ☒ FATHER ☐ MOTHER ☐ NONE ☐ GUARDIAN ☐ OTHER NAME

30. DATE NOTIF

31. CHARGE Vandalism/Shampooing in public facility, 1st DEGREE

32. ☐ FEL. ☒ MISD. ☐ INFRAC. ☐ VIOL. ☐ OFF 33. SECTION

34

35. SYNOPSIS OF FACTS
Officers called to scene greeted by sight of two figures in Flugel four
Officers approached, youths made no attempt to flee scene. Perpetrators
unable to move due to green jelly-like substance filling fountain. Back
called for when officers overcome by noxious fumes. Also arrested accompl
Theodore Nugent Fachnagel, 16 year old.

37. SLA LIC PREM. NAME(S) OF LICENSEE(S)

38. LOCATION OF INCIDENT - CITY Flugel Green, Seville BUSINESS NAME

38A. LIC NO

42. LOCATION OF ARREST - CITY Flugel Fountain

43. COUNTY NTY

36. AUTHORITY FOR ARREST
☐ PICKUP ☐ CRIM. SUMMONS ☐ WAR
☐ APPEARANCE TICKET ISSUED ☐ CITI
☐ OTHER

40. DAT

106

Perdita Buff-Smalls

"The Wounded Imago: Hair as Symbol - Sacred and Scorned"

Adapted from a talk originally presented in June 1998 at The Center for Actual Existence, Big Sur, California

From its very roots in ancient Hermetic alchemical writings to the present, the "as above, so below" dictum has found expression in myriad forms of human enterprise. Unfortunately, we have come to accept common interpretations equating the "heavenly aspects" with consciousness and the "earthbound" with the realm of the unconscious. The unconscious may as readily be seen to represent a power *above* us (often the case in dream imagery) and consciousness a realm attained by descending below.

The qualities of these polarities are embodied in the archetype of the *conjunctio*, or sacred marriage of the male and female aspects. With the notable exception of Egyptian mythology, the "above" is traditionally associated with masculine principles – i.e. order, reason, dynamism and light – and the "below" with the feminine – fertility, instinct, emotion and darkness.

In the Jungian tradition, with each archetype having a corresponding *instinct*, the *conjunctio* finds its physical expression in *sexuality*.

C A S E   S T U D Y :

A reluctant analysand was referred to me for treatment of minor depression and repeated outbursts against figures of authority. Despite his initial defensiveness and a tendency to exaggerated masculine posturing, I was immediately struck by an intrinsic innocence. This was poignantly reflected in his curious hairstyle, which was short at the top of the head (male) and long from the ears down (female). So unusual was his hair that it became the focus of several of our sessions. The subject derived considerable comfort and pride from his "Mullet," which he likened to "belonging to a brotherhood."

It would have been easy enough to dismiss this as a typically puerilistic delusion stemming from a lack of self-worth, were it not for the fact that the haircut in question was *so* compelling a physical symbol of the divine male/female union. Yet despite its power, even in a culture where traditional lines between male and female appearance and behaviors have become so blurred as to barely exist, it has not been widely embraced as such. Indeed, judging by the analysand's experiences, it seems rather to elicit feelings of *hostility* in many people (thus confirming its potency). More than any other single factor, the subject cited these repeated incidents of rejection as being at the root of his own tendency to antisocial activity.

The therapy has progressed slowly, owing in large part to the analysand's homophobic conditioning. (Any references to male/female unity, anima, etc. have had to be strictly avoided.) Yet here is a soul on the brink of psychic exhaustion who has nonetheless managed to defend and preserve his own personal expression of the *eternal embrace* against considerable odds.

That there are others like him is the *good* news. In a culture that defines the worth of its inhabitants primarily by the laws of consumerism, we need more than ever to seek the alchemical ideal. When we succeed in finding evidence of it – if only in a haircut – it is a cause for celebration, for every surviving symbol is a reminder of our inherent divinity. *[cont. page 129]*

"We know that transformation will be one of the important themes of the 21st century," writes Grant McCracken in *Big Hair: A Journey into the Transformation of Self* (1995). "Everything points in that direction.... [but] do we have a template for any of this? Do we have anything in our present experience of the world that can give us a glimpse of what lies ahead? I think we do. We can begin by taking hair seriously."

McCracken fails to consider the Mullet alongside his many examples of "big hair", but we can say with some confidence that it has always been at the forefront of the coiffureal *avant-garde*. It is a hairstyle which as much befits the cyberwarriors of the future as it does the superheroes of yesteryear, a cut that is both *of the past* and *toward the future*. Of all the styles available to modern men and women, the Mullet is surely the one best suited to the new age we are entering. If McCracken is right that, hair-wise, "we live on the edge of a great archaeological pool of possibilities", then we feel certain that the Mullet – modified and mutated – will rise swiftly to the surface.

The Cyberpudding
Two classic styles in one: this Mullet/Pudding Bowl
hybrid gives us the best of both futureworlds

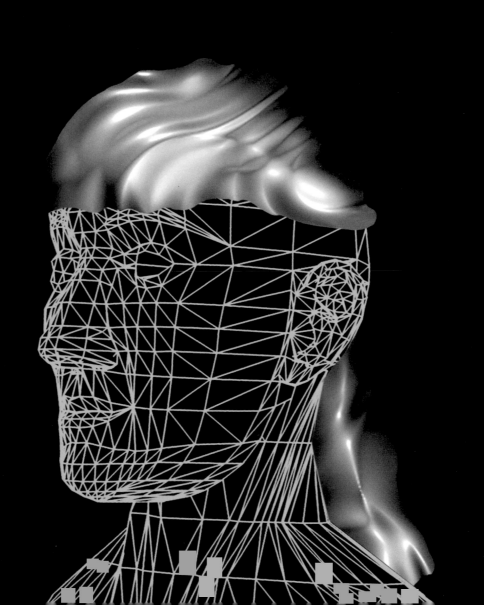

THE SCOOP

A CHIGNON STYLE THAT ROLLS FORWARD FROM THE HAIRLINE AND BACK FROM THE NAPE TO FORM A GEL-STIFFENED SPATULA

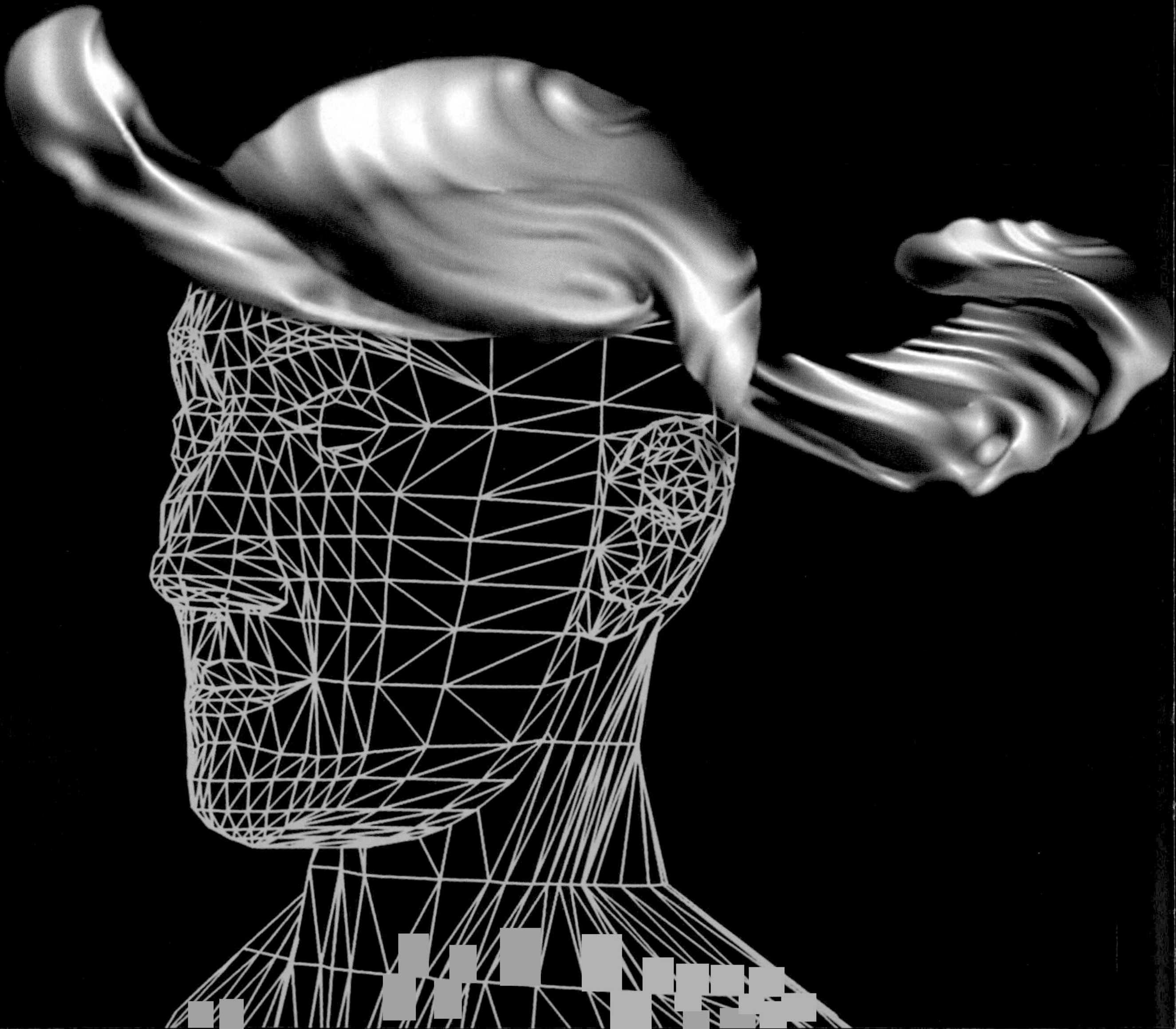

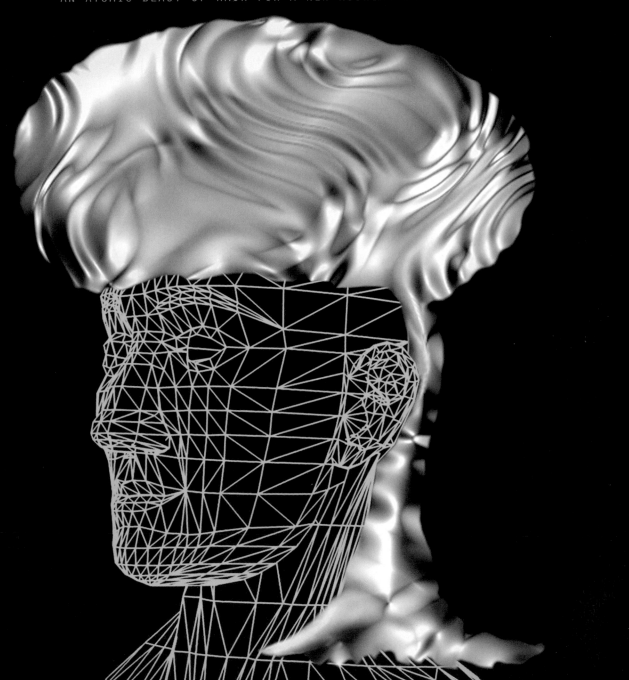

THE SHROOM
AN ATOMIC BLAST OF HAIR FOR A NEW NUCLEAR AGE

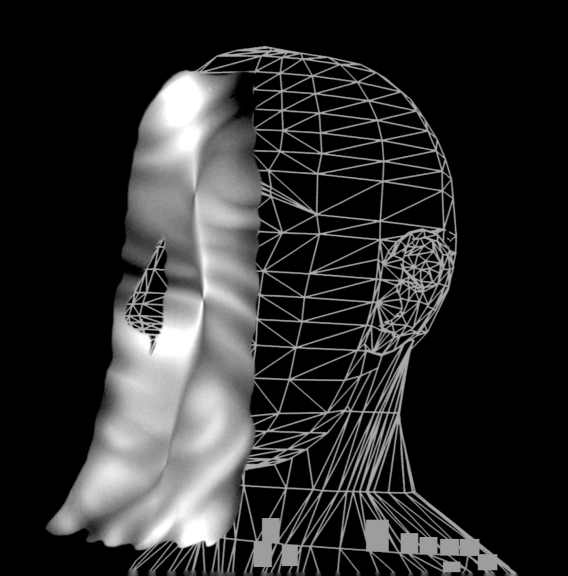

"ANGEL FALLS"
THE CLASSIC MULLET IN REVERSE, CASCADING
FROM THE FOREHEAD TO THE CHIN

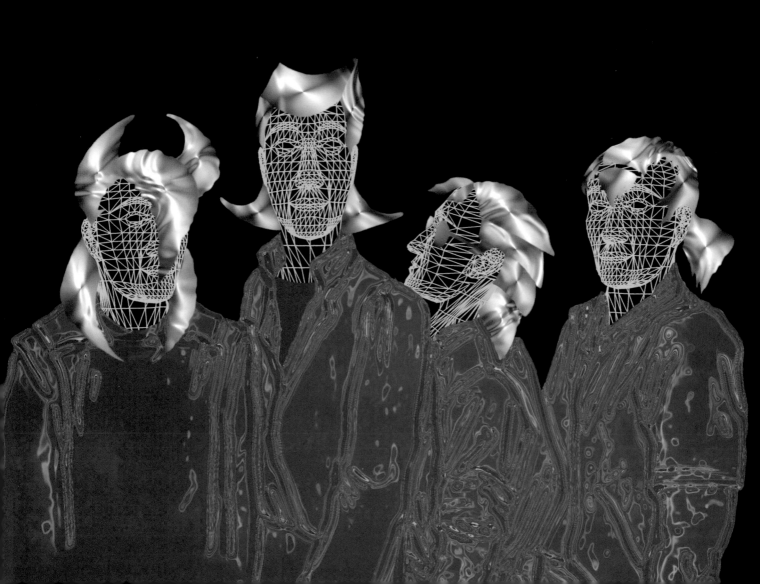

Flock o' Mullets
IN THE FUTURE THERE WILL BE TECHNO-POP GROUPS WHO LOOK
LIKE THIS. THEY WILL BE VERY COOL.

MULLETRICIDE!
Ten heinous crimes against the Mullet

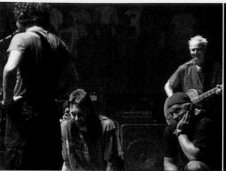 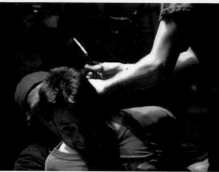 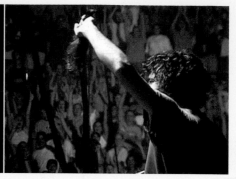

1) Mullethead Golgotha: Pearl Jam's Eddie Vedder de-Mullets a fan during a Detroit show on 23rd August, 1998. "Do you want it long or do you want it short?" demands Vedder. "Take a stand!"

2) Barbers and hairdressers who refuse to style Mullets. (They exist.)

3) David Bowie replaces his *Diamond Dogs* Mullet with the "plastic soul" hair of *Young Americans*.

4) Chris Waddle de-Mullets himself before England's 1990 World Cup semi-final against Germany and misses a vital penalty as a result.

5) The "cleansing" of Mullets from Brit uber-soap *East Enders*.

6) Christopher Moltisanti yells "Siddown, you fucking Mulletheads!" in HBO series *The Sopranos*.

7) Marc Weingarten denigrates Paul McCartney's Mullet as "hair that makes him look like an acolyte of Florence Henderson" in *Request*, September 1997 -- adding, "it's less a question of fashion etiquette than of severe mental myopia".

8) Brooke Shields claims to be "thrilled" when Andre Agassi cuts off his Mullet in 1994.

9) *Sky* Magazine's supposedly hilarious "Mullet of Justice" series, wherein assorted celebrities are "punished" by having Mullets superimposed on their heads -- blind justice!

10) The sorry lack of reference to the Lesbian Mullet in Mary Dugger's *The History of Lesbian Hair* (1996).

Also Known
A K As:
A Mullet by any other name...

the sho-lo
the camaro
the guido
the boz
the sphinx
the lobster
the mud flap
the bridge and tunnel

the bi-level
the shlong
the hockey head
the soccer rocker
the ape drape
the neck blanket
the safety cut
the long island ice tease

the kentucky waterfall
the squirrel pelt
the scorp(ion)
the butt rocker
the beaver paddle
the trans am
the south of the border
the yin and the yang
the either/or
the 10/90
the s f l b
the spooner

Call it what you want, this haircut rocks!

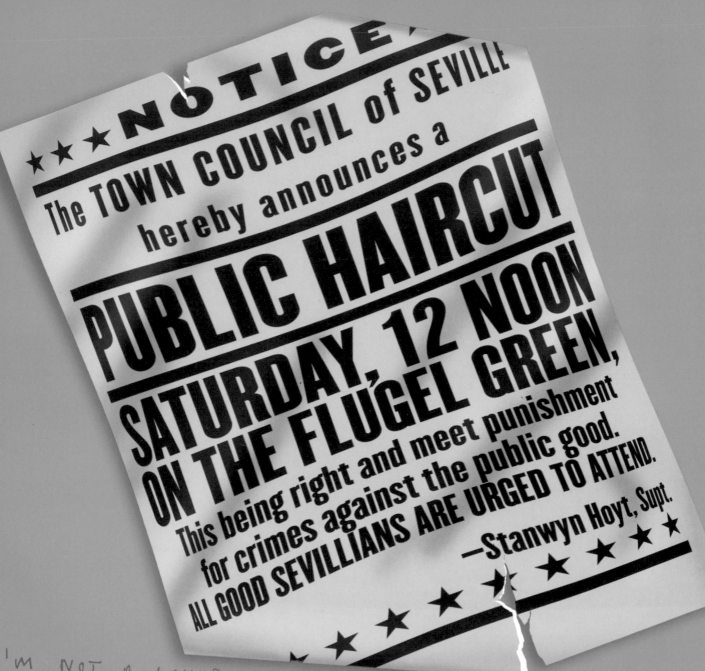

I'M NOT A LONER, I JUST END UP ALONE A LOT
- LINK P.

Mullet Kidz Korner

Ode to the Mullet
Once I woke up in my bed.
I was now a mullethead!
Then my father got one, too!
A mullet's the thing to do!
You've got to get one now!
Come on, I'll show you how!
It's such a fancy 'do!
It's the thing for me and you!

Jake (age 9)

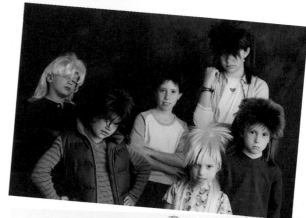

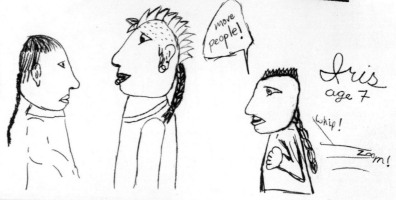

move people!

Iris
age 7

whip!

Zoom!

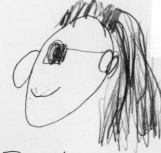

Fred (aged 6)

JUST AHEAD

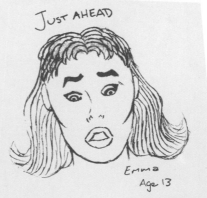

Emma
Age 13

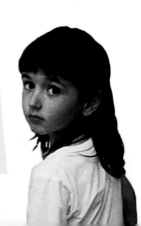

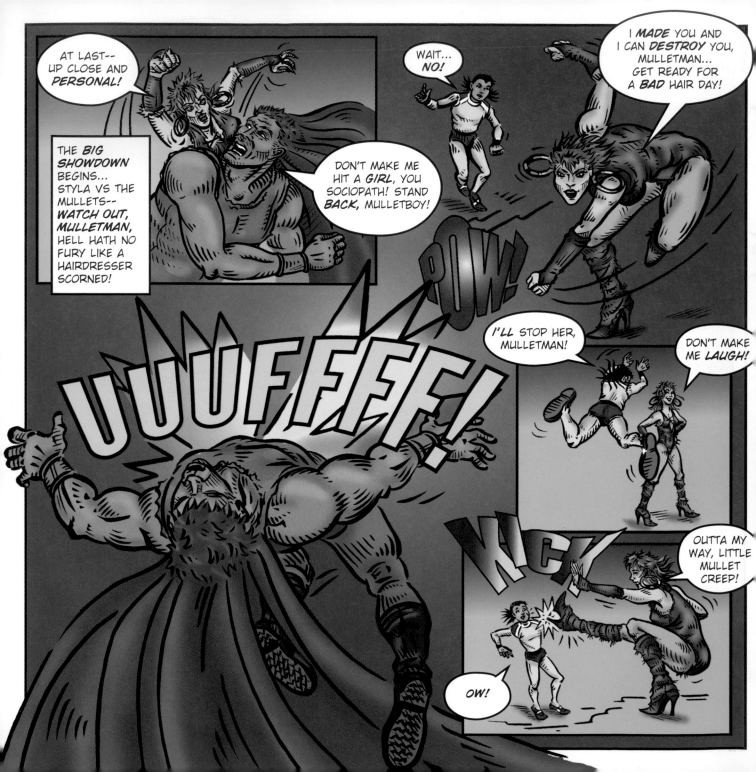

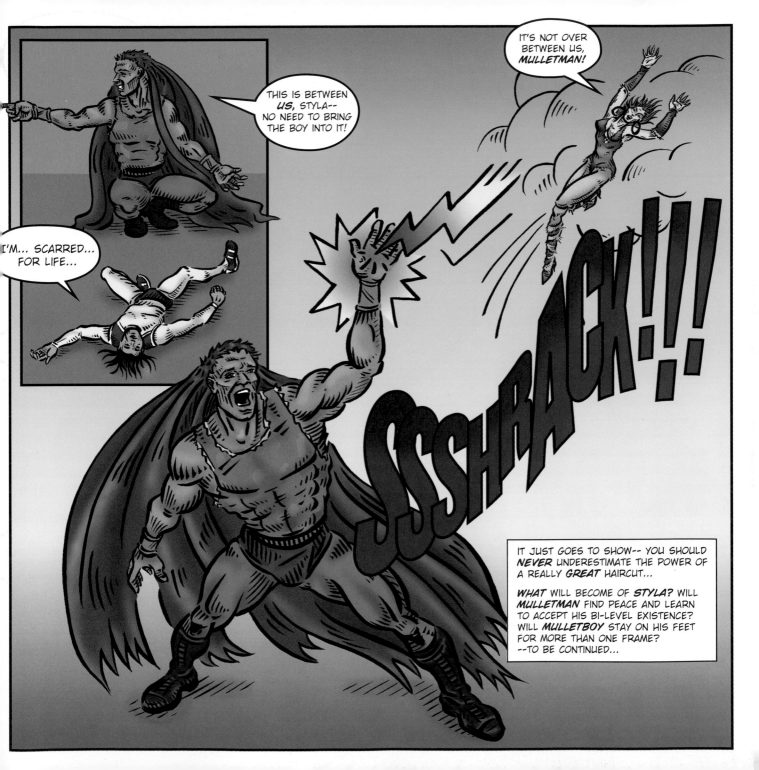

MULLET MARKETPLACE

You've read the book, now BUY the wickedly seductive merchandise!

Mullethead baseball cap:
Buy this "novelty" item for your non-Mullethead pals — they'll soon grow to love the feel of a proper "tail" dangling down their backs!

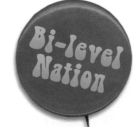

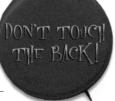

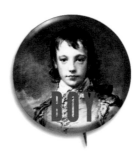

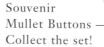

Souvenir Mullet Buttons —
Collect the set!

Mulletman action figure:
Junior 'heads will flip for this avenging action figure with the unique cape! Look for the new Mulletboy figure, coming soon!

Mulletonin: For the sweet, deep sleep every Mullethead deserves. Nurtures your locks while you snooze!

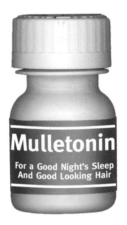

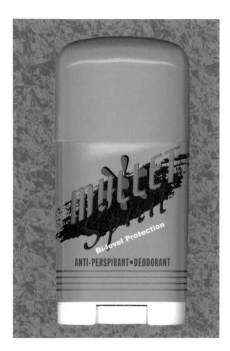

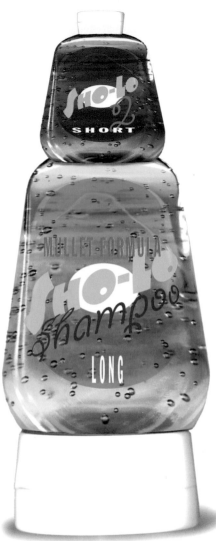

Sho-Lo Shampoo: The 2-in-1 shampoo created exclusively for Mulletheads! One treats the short hair on top, the other is for the longer stuff at the back. Now with built-in conditioner!

Mullet Spirit: "Here we are now, imitate us!" Nothing beats the deep, effective, cool-smelling protection of the Mullethead's favorite stick deodorant!

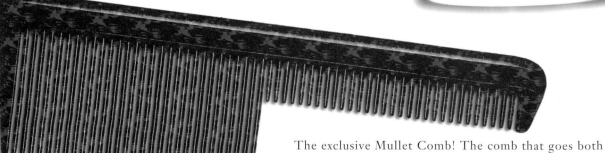

The exclusive Mullet Comb! The comb that goes both ways: short for the top & sides and long in the tooth for great Mullet back action!

SPLIT ENDS

"There will always be a new hair frontier to cross..."

Mimi Pond, *Splitting Hairs: The Bald Truth*
About Bad Hair Days (1998)

Reduced to bare physiology, hair is far from glamorous. The *American Heritage Dictionary* describes it as "cylindrical, often pigmented, filaments characteristically growing from the epidermis of a mammal". Roy Blount, Jr., in *It Grows On You: A Hair-Raising Survey of Human Plumage* (1986) is even less sentimental, calling it nothing more than "strings of deceased protein flecks, excreted by the follicles".

Put like that, it's a wonder people get so worked up about the stuff. Perhaps our obsession with our "deceased flecks" comes down to just how vulnerable they are to ridicule. As Mimi Pond writes, "our hair anxiety stems from the fact that, in this world, making fun of other people's hair is a recognized spectator sport" – a sport she terms HDA, or "Hairdo Alert". (The ultimate HDA

Mullet in flight: Mel Gibson

EXCELLENT!

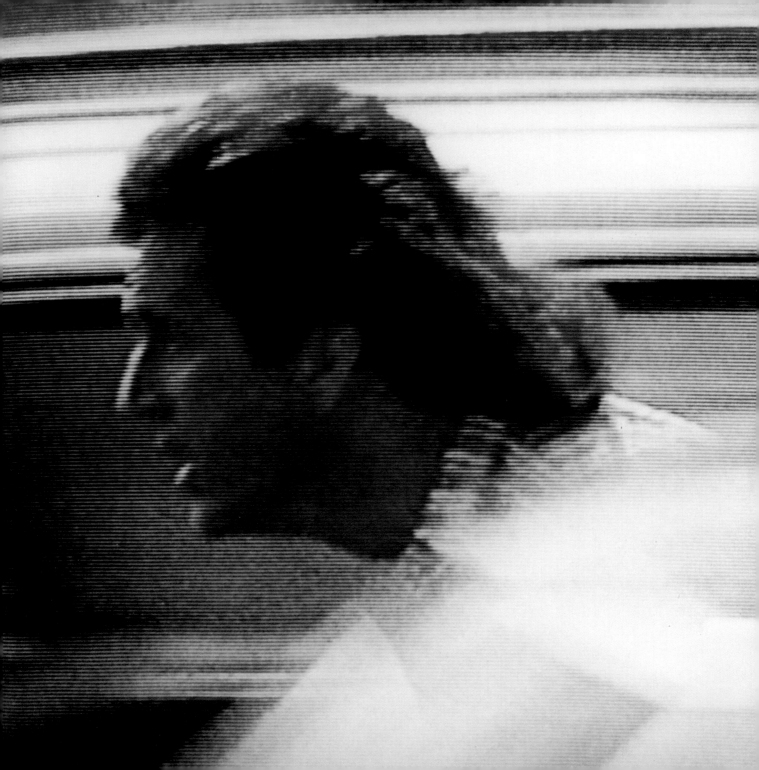

arena, she notes, is the airport, a place crammed with people "stuck for eight hours without anything to read".)

In her *Splitting Hairs*, Pond addresses the fundamental angst that accompanies hair choices in the modern world. "For some it's an endless debate; for others, no question," she writes. "Should I wear it long or short? If it's long, it may just lay there like a Portuguese man-of-war on your head, limp and slack.... [but] if it's short, is it just a copout?" Given her commendable awareness of the Mullet – her book even includes a Mullet "hair tree" with David Bowie at the roots and Billy Ray Cyrus at the top – it is odd that Pond does not consider the middle-ground solution the Mullet represents. Why, after all, should one have to choose between the long and the short of it all?

Will the Mullet ever disappear? The short answer is, not as long as people have hair and ears. Asked in 1998 if "an '80s revival could once more make the Mullet a viable hair option", the Beastie Boys' Adam Yauch replied, quite rightly, that the Mullet was "not a specific thing of the '80s... it has such a huge history". (During the World Cup that year, sports fans the world over were treated to the spectacular Soccer Mullet of South Korean goalkeeper Kim. Sadly, Kim's coiffure was not enough to

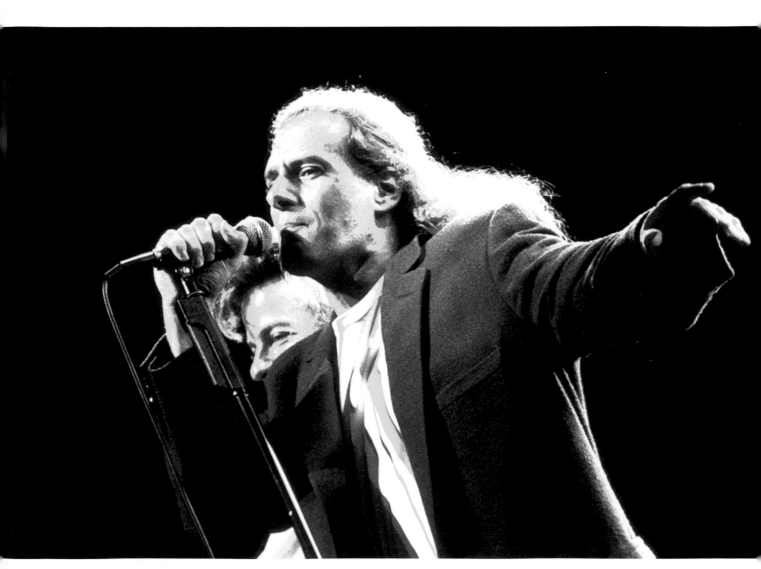

Mullet in flight II: Michael Bolton

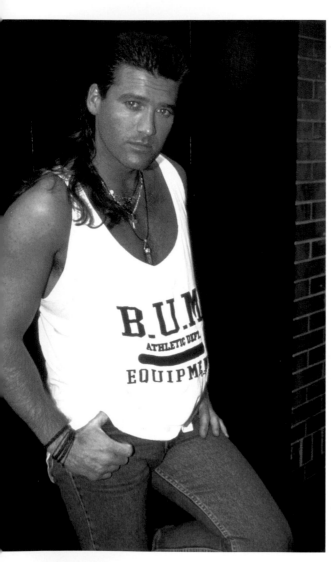

Mullet in repose: the incomparable Mr. Cyrus

stop Dutch, Belgian, and Mexican strikers putting ten goals past him, thus eliminating his country from the tournament.)

"Mullethead society has developed into what it is today, a worldwide organization of individuals who use intricate handshakes, songs and phrases to keep traditions alive, and to provide hours of entertainment to non-Mulletheads." So wrote the members of Hot Stove Jimmy, a ten-piece Chicago band who – with no government funding – spent a goodly portion of the 1990s researching the Great American Mullet.

On one of Hot Stove Jimmy's "Mullet Research Expeditions", in 1997, the band pulled into a truck stop in Maryland. Here, as noted on their Website, they had the singular pleasure of beholding an "extremely rare and elusive" Asian Mullet. No, it wasn't South Korea's goalkeeper but a young female with "a light feathery flow" who "sifted methodically through the $3.99 bin of discount tapes offering titles by such artists as Cinderella, Judas Priest, White Lion, and Twisted Sister". When the Fe-Mullethead in question sensed the group's collective presence, she "quickly scurried off and disappeared somewhere between the pork rinds and the Marlboro racing team cardboard cutout".

Let us trust that further field research will not scare such creatures into disappearing altogether. In Thomas Frank's words, the Mullet is a hairstyle that dwells in "the shadow of irony". We feel confident that its adherents will always be proud to let it flow in the broad light of day.

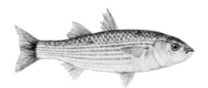

EAT MY TAIL!

"Stare long enough into the Mullet
and it will stare back into you."

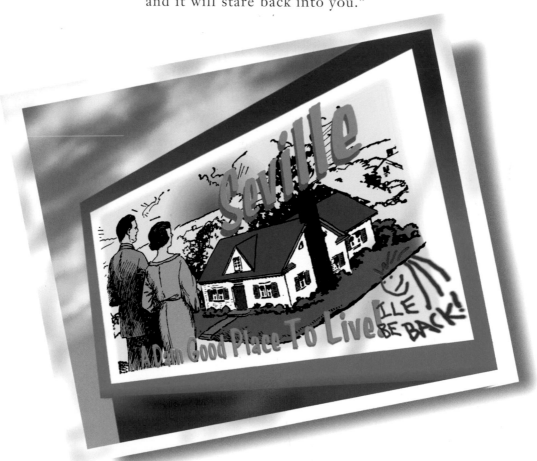